NUFFIELD
COUNCIL ON
BIOETHICS

Animal-to-Human Transplants

the ethics of xenotransplantation

Nuffield Council on Bioethics

The terms of reference are as follows:

1 to identify and define ethical questions raised by recent advances in biological and medical research in order to respond to, and to anticipate, public concern;

2 to make arrangements for examining and reporting on such questions with a view to promoting public understanding and discussion; this may lead, where needed, to the formulation of new guidelines by the appropriate regulatory or other body; and

3 in the light of the outcome of its work, to publish reports; and to make representations, as the Council may judge appropriate.

The Nuffield Council on Bioethics is funded jointly by the Medical Research Council, the Nuffield Foundation and the Wellcome Trust

Preface

Since the Nuffield Council on Bioethics decided to initiate an inquiry into xenotransplantation (animal-to-human transplants), the issues posed by that clinical procedure have become more important and urgent in the light of:

- the continuing shortfall of human donation to meet the growing demand for organ transplantation;
- growing uncertainty about the risk of the potential transmission of diseases by xenografts;
- public concern about the proper use of the genetic modification of animals;
- wide and increasing concern about animal welfare.

In the United Kingdom these concerns have been highlighted by the announcement in September 1995 by the UK company Imutran Ltd that, in the light of its research with pigs and monkeys, it envisaged the first xenografts of transgenic pig hearts into human patients taking place in 1996.

The Council set up a Working Party in January 1995 under the chairmanship of Professor Albert Weale. The Working Party engaged in a wide public consultation. Its report has now been carefully considered and endorsed by the Council. Its importance has been underlined by the Government decision last September to set up a committee of its own, chaired by Professor Ian Kennedy (a member of the Nuffield Council on Bioethics), which is also examining xenotransplantation. That committee can be expected to draw on and complement this report.

The report sets out the progress made in developing xenotransplantation as a procedure, and it addresses a range of key questions. What effective alternatives exist? Is it ethically acceptable to use animals for this purpose - specifically primates and transgenic pigs? Will xenografts be safe? How will patients react? What are the implications for the NHS?

The principal conclusions and recommendations are these:

- there is a prospect that xenotransplantation may be able to supplement significantly the present inadequate supply of human organs - both to save life and to improve the quality of life; but complex questions of ethics and serious problems of safety need to be resolved;

- in view of the potential benefit to patients, whose needs cannot at present be effectively met in other ways, the breeding of pigs to supply organs for xenotransplantation would be ethically justified. There are strong reasons for using pigs rather than higher primates for this purpose;

- there is an immediate need to establish an Advisory Committee on Xenotransplantation for the purpose of assessing the potential public health risks from infectious organisms of animals; establishing the essential precautionary measures prior to any clinical human trials; and protecting the interests of the patients who receive xenografts;

- once all the necessary safeguards have been set in place, xenotransplantation may be offered to suitable patients. Strict ethical procedures relating to consent should be followed, and patients unwilling to consent to xenotransplantation should not be disadvantaged in any way. Should xenotransplantation become introduced into clinical practice, its impact on individual patients should be the subject of research.

The Council hopes that the conclusions and recommendations of this report will be fully considered by the Government, and by the professional and other bodies and the commercial organisations concerned. There remains an urgent need to increase the scale of donation of human organs; but, even if that were achieved, a safe and acceptable programme of xenotransplantation may be of great value in the benefit it could offer to many additional patients. To that end it is hoped that the report will stimulate immediate and wide public interest and discussion.

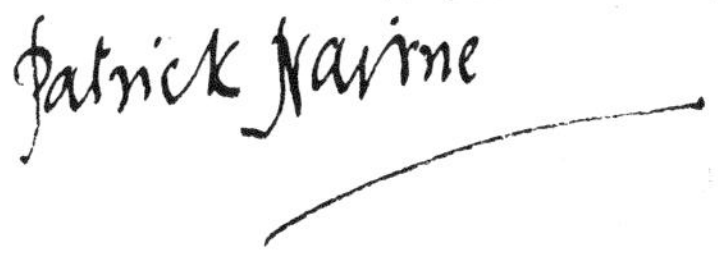

Rt Hon **Sir Patrick Nairne** GCB MC
Chairman
Nuffield Council on Bioethics

Table of contents

Working Party on Xenografts

Professor **Albert Weale**, Chairman
Professor of Government at the University of Essex

Ms **Virginia Beardshaw** is Director of Commissioning at Barnet Health Agency

Dr **Roger Crisp** is Fellow and Tutor in Philosophy at St Anne's College, Oxford

Professor **Celia Davies** is Professor of Health Care at the Open University

Ms **Annabel Ferriman** is a freelance medical journalist

Professor **Tim Ingold** is Professor of Social Anthropology at the University of Manchester

Professor **John Ledingham** was formerly Professor of Clinical Medicine, University of Oxford, John Radcliffe Hospital

Professor **David Morton** is a veterinary surgeon and Professor of Biomedical Science and Biomedical Ethics at the University of Birmingham

Dr **Brian Newbould** is a member of the Nuffield Council on Bioethics and was formerly Director of International Research Affairs, ICI Corporate Research and Technology

Professor **Mark Walport** is a Professor of Medicine at the Royal Postgraduate Medical School, Hammersmith Hospital, London

Secretariat
Dr Rachel Bartlett
Mrs Jill Batty
Mr David Shapiro

Working Party on Xenografts

Terms of Reference

1 To review recent and prospective advances in xenografts and the current and prospective applications of such procedures. For these purposes xenografts are defined as the transplantation of animal cells, tissues or organs into human beings.

2 To identify and consider the ethical issues arising from current and prospective uses of xenografts, including in particular:

a the ethical aspects of the case for xenografts in the light of alternative procedures or practices, taking into account current and potential benefits and current and potential difficulties;

b the use of animals as sources of cells, tissues or organs;

c the special care and maintenance of the animals intended for that use;

d the ethical implications of transferring human genes into animals to allow the subsequent transplantation of animal cells, tissues or organs into human beings,

e any other ethical issues arising from experimentation with transgenic animals to enable their use as sources of xenografts - taking account, in particular, of the possibilities of the transmission of disease across species boundaries.

Summary of recommendations

Xenotransplantation raises a particularly wide range of concerns about which people have differing and strongly held views. The Working Party has concluded that the development of xenotransplantation should continue subject to rigorous regulation to ensure protection for potential human recipients and care for animal welfare. The recommendations of the Working Party are as follows:

Animal concerns: principles

1 The Working Party endorses the special protection afforded to primates used for medical and scientific purposes (paragraph 10.9). Non-primate species should be regarded as the source animals of choice for xenotransplantation (paragraph 10.12).

2 The use of pigs for the routine supply of organs for xenotransplantation is ethically acceptable (paragraph 10.14). The use of transgenic pigs that have been genetically modified to reduce the human immune response to pig organs is also ethically acceptable (paragraph 10.15).

Animal concerns: practice

3 The Home Office should require that all animals used for xenotransplantation are protected under the Animals (Scientific Procedures) Act 1986 (paragraph 10.23). Thus, the standards set by the 1986 Act should become the minimum for the industry (paragraph 10.23). The convention by which the Animal Procedures Committee advises on project licences in difficult areas should extend to applications for the use of animals for xenotransplantation (paragraph 10.18).

4 When decisions are made about the acceptability of using animals for xenotransplantation, particular attention should be paid to reducing the adverse effects associated with the need to produce animals free from infectious organisms (paragraph 10.21). The Animals (Scientific Procedures) Act should continue to be interpreted as prohibiting sequential removal from animals of tissues or organs for transplantation (paragraph 10.22).

Transmission of infectious diseases

5 The risks associated with possible transmission of infectious diseases as a consequence of xenotransplantation have not been adequately dealt with. It would not be ethical therefore to begin clinical trials of xenotransplantation involving human beings (paragraph 10.25).

6 A code of practice should be drawn up specifying which organisms should be excluded from specified-pathogen free animals. Xenotransplantation teams should be required to exclude from source animals all the pathogens listed in the code of practice (paragraph 10.27). A regulatory framework should be devised to control the safety and quality of animal organs and tissue for xenotransplantation (paragraph 10.27).

7 Standards and mechanisms for monitoring xenograft recipients and for the action to be taken in case of disease transmission should be in place before human trials begin. It should be a requirement of clinical trials that the need for monitoring is explained to the patient and that it is made clear that consent to the operation also implies consent to subsequent monitoring (paragraph 10.28). Xenotransplantation teams should be required to record all information concerning individual xenograft recipients in a xenotransplantation register maintained by an independent body (paragraph 10.29).

8 The Working Party recommends that the Department of Health should establish an Advisory Committee on Xenotransplantation (paragraph 10.31).

Early patients

9 No xenotransplantation trials involving human recipients should proceed until the proposed Advisory Committee on Xenotransplantation is in place and has approved the trials (paragraph 10.32). Consent of patients to participation in xenotransplantation trials should be sought by appropriately trained professionals who are independent of the xenotransplantation team. The information given to prospective recipients should include an estimation of likely success, attendant risks and subsequent quality of life (paragraph 10.34). No protocol to conduct a trial should be accepted unless it contains a commitment to a robust description and assessment of the patient's pre-operative and post-operative quality of life (paragraph 10.35).

10 The first xenotransplantation trials should involve adults rather than children (paragraph 10.36). The first xenotransplantation trials should not involve adults incapable of consenting to participation on their own behalf (paragraph 10.38).

11 At any stage in the development of xenotransplantation, patients who, for whatever reasons, refuse xenografts should remain entitled to consideration for human organs on the same basis as before their refusal (paragraph 10.40). Xenograft recipients should remain entitled to consideration for human organ transplantation on the same basis of clinical need as before xenotransplantation (paragraph 10.41).

Effects on the health care system

12 If xenotransplantation becomes a treatment of choice, the introduction of the treatment into the NHS should be overseen by the Supra Regional Services Advisory Group (paragraph 10.43).

Personal and social effects of xenotransplantation

13 Counselling of xenograft recipients should include discussion of the possible personal impact of xenotransplantation. Research should be initiated to assess the personal impact of xenotransplantation on potential and early recipients (paragraph 10.45).

Implementation of recommendations

14 The Working Party recommends that the proposed Advisory Committee on Xenotransplantation should produce guidance on best practice and revise that guidance in the light of experience. The responsibilities of the Advisory Committee should include (paragraph 10.47):

- assembling and assessing information about the possible risks of disease transmission, and on that basis making recommendations (paragraph 10.26)
- establishing a regulatory mechanism to ensure that the appropriate infectious organisms are eliminated from source animals (paragraph 10.27)
- developing guidance on the monitoring of future recipients of xenografts and maintaining a register of xenograft recipients (paragraphs 10.28 - 10.29)
- approving any xenotransplantation trials involving human recipients and the centres that may undertake such trials (paragraph 10.32)
- overseeing issues of consent and conscientious objection (paragraphs 10.34 - 10.41)
- assessing the impact of xenotransplantation on individual recipients (paragraph 10.45)
- facilitating debate and assessing attitudes to xenotransplantation (paragraph 10.46).

No xenotransplantation trials involving human recipients should proceed until the proposed Advisory Committee on Xenotransplantation is in place and the above issues have been addressed.

Animal-to-Human Transplants

the ethics of xenotransplantation

Chapter 1

The promise and the problems

1.1 Rare attempts have been made to transplant animal organs or tissue into human beings since the early years of this century. Interest in this procedure, known as xenotransplantation, has increased in the last few years because it is seen as one way of reducing the shortage of human organs for transplantation. Currently, this shortage severely limits the potential of transplantation for treating human disease.

1.2 The prospect of using animal organs and tissue for xenotransplantation raises important issues, both practical and ethical, which must be debated. Will xenotransplantation be scientifically feasible? If so, should it be permitted? Are there safety risks for recipients, or for the public at large? If so, how can patients and the wider population be protected? Should animals be used in this way? This chapter sets out the main issues raised by xenotransplantation to be discussed in the body of the report. First, however, it sets the scene by describing the increasing success of transplantation for treating organ failure and other conditions, and the increasingly acute shortage of human organs and tissue for transplantation.

Transplantation in medicine

1.3 For many conditions involving organ failure, transplantation has become routine, and is often the treatment of choice. In the early days, problems with organ rejection, and infections resulting from early immunosuppressive regimes, made transplantation a risky procedure. But a new generation of immunosuppressive drugs, and improved surgical techniques, now allow patients to receive transplants relatively safely and with considerable benefit. As Table 1.1 shows, more than four in five kidney transplant recipients live for at least a year, and over two-thirds live for at least five years. Other transplants are not as successful, but even in the least successful case of liver transplants, more than half the recipients live for longer than five years.

Table 1.1 One year and five year survival rates of transplant recipients[1]

Organ	Survival Rates	
	1 year	5 years
Kidney	84%	70%
Liver	62%	54%
Heart	73%	62%

1.4 Organ transplantation offers several benefits. For some conditions, such as advanced heart failure, treatment with drugs or restorative surgery may not be possible and a transplant will provide the only way of replacing a failed vital organ. Heart or liver transplantation can offer many additional years of life for people who otherwise might not survive, as the one year and five year survival rates for liver and heart transplant recipients show (Table 1.1). Worldwide there are patients whose lives have been considerably extended following transplantation: by 23 years after liver transplants and 20 years after heart transplants.

1.5 Transplantation can not only increase the length of life, but also improve its quality. Even where there is an alternative form of treatment, such as dialysis for end-stage kidney failure, a transplant frequently offers a higher quality of life despite the drawbacks of the continuous immunosuppressive regime most transplant recipients require. Kidney transplant recipients are freed from the necessity of regular, uncomfortable and time-consuming treatment and are restored to a level of health not possible with dialysis. They are able to eat and drink freely, and to travel, in ways that people on long-term dialysis often cannot. Patient support groups describe heart transplant recipients who are able to climb hills, and undertake other activities, that they would not have been able to manage before the operation. Some transplant recipients participate in highly demanding sporting contests such as the Transplant Games.

1.6 It should be noted that, contrary to some misperception, transplantation is not particularly expensive. Estimates are very difficult to make, but it is possible to get a rough idea of the relative costs of different treatments. A kidney transplant operation costs in the region of £10,000. After that, the cost of immunosuppressive drugs and other follow-up treatment is about £3,000 a year. In contrast, dialysis costs about £18,000 a year if the patient is treated in hospital, and about £11,000 if the patient is treated at home. Thus, kidney transplantation is a more cost-effective

---

1 Source: United Kingdom Transplant Support Service Authority (UKTSSA) publications: **Renal Transplant Audit 1984-1993; Liver Transplant Audit 1985-1992; Thoracic Organ Transplant Audit 1985-1992.**

treatment for patients with renal failure than long-term dialysis. The cost of other transplant operations varies according to how long the patient remains in hospital. Heart transplants cost about £10,000 - £18,000 and liver transplants about £15,000 - £18,000. Immunosuppressive drugs and other follow-up treatment after a liver transplant cost about £3,000 - £5,000 a year.[2]

The demand for organs

1.7 The success of transplantation, however, brings with it the problem of obtaining an adequate supply of human organs for such treatments. In the UK, the majority of human organs for transplantation come from donors who are brain stem dead but whose lungs are being artificially ventilated in an intensive care unit and whose hearts are still beating. Most of these people have suffered severe brain damage, mainly caused by brain haemorrhages or road accidents. Some organs, such as kidneys, can be removed from donors whose hearts are no longer beating. And kidneys, sections of the liver, and some tissues such as bone marrow, can be donated by living people. Live donation, however, is a major procedure and it is not possible for hearts. Thus, the supply of organs for transplantation is very restricted and falls far short of demand. Even if all human cadaveric organs were somehow made available for transplant, the supply would still not meet the potential demand.[3] Meanwhile, as the benefits of transplantation have become more apparent, so the demand for this form of treatment has increased and the shortage of human organs has become more acute. This is illustrated by the figures for kidney transplantation, the most commonly performed transplant operation (Figure 1.1). In 1978, in the UK and the Republic of Ireland, 765 kidney transplant operations were performed, and 1,274 people remained on the waiting list. By 1994, the number of transplants performed that year had increased to 1,744, but the number of people remaining on the waiting list had increased to 4,970.[4]

---

2 Another method of estimating treatment costs uses the QALY or Quality Adjusted Life Year, which tries to take account of the increase in life-expectancy and quality of life gained by treatment. This method has its difficulties, but it can give a rough idea of treatment costs. It indicates, for example, that a kidney transplant is about four times more expensive than a hip replacement, but confirms that it is a less expensive treatment for kidney failure than dialysis (Mason J *et al.* (1993) Some guidelines on the use of cost effectiveness league tables. **British Medical Journal**, 306:570-2).

3 Caplan A (1992) Is xenografting morally wrong? **Transplantation Proceedings**, 24:722-7, quoted in Tania Woods' submission to the Working Party.

4 United Kingdom Transplant Support Service Authority (UKTSSA) (1995) Yearly transplant statistics for the United Kingdom and Republic of Ireland as notified to UKTSSA. UKTSSA information sheet.

Figure 1.1 **Number of kidney transplants and size of waiting list**[5]

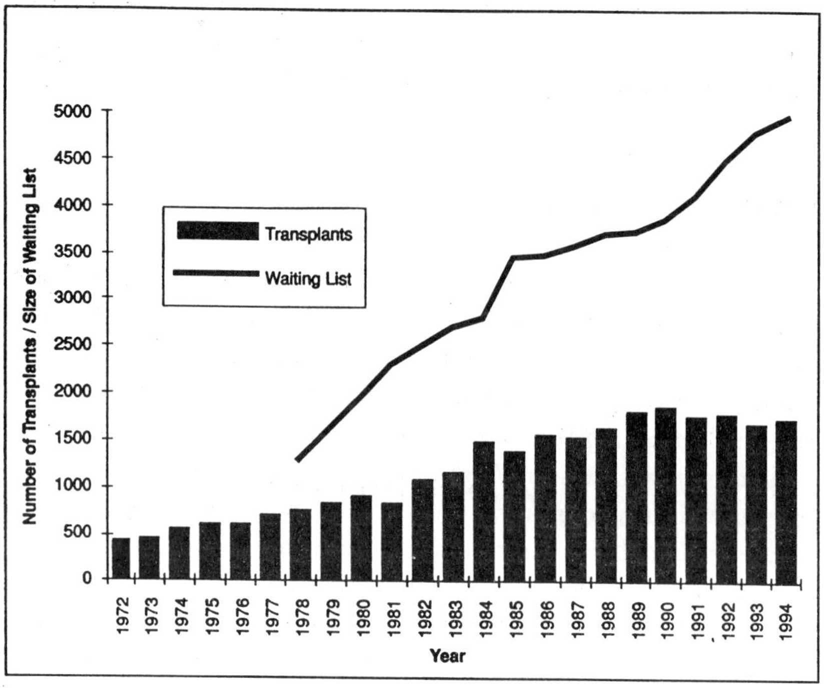

1.8 Fewer heart transplants are performed, but the organ shortage is still acute: in 1994, 328 transplants were performed, but 320 patients remained on the waiting list.[6] Unlike patients with kidney failure, who can receive dialysis, patients with end-stage heart failure often have no alternative form of effective treatment and many will die while waiting for a suitable donor organ. This means that the length of the waiting list underestimates the demand for heart transplants. In addition, the organ shortage means that the criteria for eligibility for transplantation are very strict: organs are transplanted into those for whom there is the most pressing need and the best chance that the operation will be successful. Many people who might benefit from a transplant if more organs were available never make it onto the waiting list for human organs. It is estimated that, if sufficient organs were available, the number of people in the UK who could benefit from heart transplantation would be five times the number that can currently hope to receive an organ.[7] Since the incidence of heart failure increases with age, as the number of elderly people in the UK increases, the demand for heart transplants is likely to increase still further.

5 Figure reproduced with kind permission from UKTSSA information sheet (1995). Figures are for cadaveric kidney transplants.

6 UKTSSA information sheet (1995).

7 Westaby S (1996) The need for artificial hearts. **British Heart Journal,** in press.

1.9 It is not only organs, such as the kidneys, heart, liver and lung, which are transplanted, but also human tissue and cells. Hip replacements may involve transplants of bone and treatment of burns may require skin transplants. Less common is the transplantation of neural tissue for treating Parkinson's disease and the transplantation of pancreatic islet cells for treating diabetes. The shortage of human organs is especially pressing, since they are usually required to treat otherwise terminal diseases that cannot be treated in any other way. In contrast, there may be alternatives to treating a condition if tissue is not available for transplantation, and the condition itself may not be so life-threatening. Moreover, much human tissue, like bone and skin, can regenerate and can, therefore, be obtained from living donors. Nevertheless, in addition to the difficulty of obtaining organs, there are also difficulties in obtaining supplies of human tissue and cells for transplantation. Further developments in transplantation are likely to lead to its use for treating a wider range of conditions and so to increased demand for human material for transplantation.

Reducing the shortage of human organs

1.10 How can the shortfall between the supply of, and the demand for, human organs and tissue be overcome? One approach is to try and reduce the demand through preventive measures to improve health: at present some transplants are required for conditions that should be avoidable. Another approach is to introduce measures to improve the supply of human organs and tissue. It is often suggested that, if the UK adopted measures similar to countries with a higher transplantation rate, it could increase its transplant activity. As discussed in Chapter 2, however, changing policy to improve human organ supply is a sensitive issue. In addition, certain factors affecting transplantation rates may be beyond the control of policy changes. In the UK, for example, the low number of organ donors is due in part to the wholly desirable decline in deaths due to road traffic accidents or brain haemorrhage.[8, 9]

1.11 Another possibility for reducing the human organ shortage is to develop artificial replacements for organs and tissue. These may be mechanical devices, like the battery-powered heart, or bioengineered structures incorporating human or animal material. Many of these developments hold promise for the future but, as discussed in Chapter 2, they remain problematic for the time being.

---

8 New B *et al.* (1994) **A Question of Give and Take: Improving the supply of donor organs for transplantation.** King's Fund Institute Research Report 18.

9 **Report of the British Transplantation Society Working Party on Organ Donation** (1995) British Transplantation Society.

The promise of xenotransplantation

1.12 The demand for human organs and tissue for transplantation exceeds their availability and the gap between supply and demand is likely to increase (Chapter 2). In these circumstances one possibility is that the imbalance could be redressed by using other animals as sources of material for transplantation into human beings. Pig heart valves have been used in human heart surgery for 30 years. Attempts to transplant animal organs into human beings are far more ambitious. To date this has not been successful. The best result was recorded in the case of one patient who lived for nine months in the 1960s having received a transplanted chimpanzee's kidney.

1.13 The major hurdle in the way of successful xenotransplantation is preventing the rejection of transplanted animal organs. This is a problem even with human organ transplantation: the recipient's immune system mounts an attack on the transplanted organ, which it sees as foreign. The immune response to organs or tissue from a different species is much stronger. Two main approaches are being used to overcome this problem. First, in the United States, the use of baboons is being investigated, on the basis that baboons are closely related to human beings and so the immune response to baboon organs or tissue will not be too strong. The second approach is to use pigs that have been modified genetically so that their organs do not cause such a strong immune response when transplanted into human beings. These two approaches are described in more detail in Chapter 3.

1.14 Xenotransplantation offers promise, not only for organ transplantation, but also for the transplantation of tissue and cells. Xenotransplantation of animal bone, skin, bone marrow, pancreatic islet cells, and fetal neural tissue have all been suggested. Xenotransplantation of tissue is a less drastic procedure than organ xenotransplantation. The immune response is less vigorous for small pieces of tissue which do not have a major blood supply running through them and the surgical procedure is likely to be less risky. The impact on the recipient may also be less severe since it seems that people attach more significance to organ transplantation than to the transplantation of tissue or cells. Moreover, as mentioned above, it is the shortage of human organs that is particularly acute. For this reason, the discussion in this report will largely concern the xenotransplantation of organs. Much of what is said about organs, however, will also apply to xenotransplantation of tissue and cells. Where xenotransplantation of tissue or cells raises particular issues, these have been discussed. The transfer of molecules between species lies outside the scope of the report (paragraph 3.8).

1.15 Recent developments suggest that xenotransplantation teams are making progress in controlling the immune response to animal transplants in order to prevent rejection. Even if this becomes possible, there is also the question of whether animal organs and tissue will be able to perform all the necessary functions in a human body.

Nevertheless, it is looking increasingly probable that many of the biological obstacles to xenotransplantation will eventually be overcome.

1.16 Proponents of xenotransplantation argue that there would be significant benefits if it were to become a successful and widely available treatment. Most importantly, enough animals could be reared to provide sufficient organs and tissue to overcome the present shortage of human organs and tissue for transplantation. This would eliminate the decline in health, the considerable anxieties, and the loss of life associated with the current long waits for human organs and tissue. Instead, xenografts could be offered as and when they were needed. Xenografts could also be offered to a wider group of patients who might benefit from transplantation but who are currently not eligible for a human organ or tissue transplant. Successful xenotransplantation of genetically modified organs and tissue would also eliminate the need for the careful matching of the organ or tissue with the recipient, required in transplants between human beings in order to reduce rejection by the immune system. This would be of particular benefit to people for whom it is currently more difficult to find compatible organs and tissue: for example, people from ethnic minorities for whom there is a shortage of donors with the same or similar tissue type.

1.17 Xenotransplantation would also avoid the need to consult the relatives of dead people about organ donation at times of great stress and emotional turmoil. If there are alternative sources of organs, it will not be necessary for relatives to make such difficult decisions. The need to perform transplant operations at very short notice, as occurs when human organs become available, would also be avoided: patients and health care workers could prepare themselves for the operation in advance. Transplantation would become an easier service to coordinate and administer, and this might bring savings in cost.

1.18 For some, xenotransplantation would be preferable to some of the current or proposed methods of obtaining human organs and tissue. Despite legislation in many countries prohibiting this, the buying and selling of human organs, especially kidneys, continues.[10] If xenotransplantation were successful in reducing the shortage of organs and tissue, such ethically unacceptable commercial dealings might stop. Proponents of xenotransplantation have pointed out that, in addition, it might provide an alternative to the use of human tissue from aborted fetuses, and to methods for obtaining human organs such as elective ventilation or live donation, all of which have their difficulties (Chapter 2). However, xenotransplantation itself raises important and wide-ranging ethical concerns which need to be addressed before a judgement can be made about its acceptability. The range of these concerns is set out below.

---

10 Arguments against commercial dealings in human tissue were set out in a previous report of the Nuffield Council on Bioethics (1995) **Human Tissue : Ethical and Legal Issues.**

Ethical concerns

1.19 Xenotransplantation raises the question of how far, if at all, and in what ways it is acceptable for human beings to use other animals as a source of organs and tissue for transplantation. Even if one accepts in principle the use of animals in medicine and in medical research, their use in xenotransplantation may raise particular difficulties. The use of primates such as baboons would concern many. The use of genetically modified animals, which is likely to be necessary if pigs are to be used for xenotransplantation, also merits special consideration. And if the use of animals to supply organs for xenotransplantation is considered ethically acceptable in principle, can the welfare of the animals be adequately taken into account? These and other issues are discussed in Chapters 4 and 5.

1.20 Public health issues arise from the prospect of xenotransplantation. The transplantation of animal organs or tissue raises the possibility that infectious organisms of animals may be transferred into the human population. Xenotransplantation, like any major innovation, may have wide-ranging and unpredictable effects. It is necessary, therefore, to identify principles which would provide a basis for dealing with the remote, and unquantifiable, hazards that xenotransplantation could bring. This is discussed in Chapter 6.

1.21 The treatment of early recipients of xenografts may raise serious ethical issues. So far the survival times for recipients of xenografts have been poor and, in effect, early recipients are being used as experimental subjects for the development of the technology (Table 3.1). The principles that should govern early clinical trials for xenotransplantation are discussed in Chapter 7.

1.22 Widespread introduction of xenotransplantation could have implications for the health care system. There will be cost implications, particularly in a cash limited health care system like that of the UK. It is possible that xenotransplantation would displace other, perhaps more worthwhile, activities. The cost implications of xenotransplantation, and how the health service might control the introduction of xenotransplantation, is considered in Chapter 8.

1.23 Xenotransplantation may also have social implications. It needs to be assessed in the context of the wider debate about modern medicine and attempts to prolong life. Possible personal effects of xenotransplantation on those who are recipients need to be considered. It is impossible to say in advance what form and intensity these will take. Finally, it is important to consider how the use of animals as sources of organs might affect people's willingness to donate organs. These issues are discussed in Chapter 9.

1.24 The extent and importance of these ethical issues raises the question whether existing regulatory structures are adequate for managing the development of xenotransplantation. In Chapter 10 the different strands of the discussion are drawn together and suggestions are made for the appropriate regulation of xenotransplantation. The Working Party considers that the range of issues raised by xenotransplantation and the potential consequences of its practice are so great that there is a need for a national body to keep developments constantly under review.

The importance of moral convictions

1.25 In considering the ethical issues raised by xenotransplantation, great emphasis was placed by the Working Party on the importance of the moral convictions that people hold. It is sometimes argued that ethics and morality can be distinguished. According to this argument, codes of ethics are seen as derived by a process of abstract reasoning from first principles that are timeless and universal. Morality, by contrast, is seen as a set of rules, norms and expectations, specific to a particular culture and a particular time, which rests on tradition, sentiment and sympathy. Even where ethical systems prescribe respect for the beliefs of ordinary people, the rationality of those beliefs is often questioned.

1.26 Ethical deliberation does not take place in a vacuum, however, but in a social and historical context that is continually changing. There are no timeless solutions, and ethical debate cannot be separated from the domain of social life. Equally, people's moral convictions are not just rooted in the force of tradition but are the results of sincere and mature reflection. This was reflected in the submissions received by the Working Party on the subject of xenotransplantation.

1.27 Wherever people are involved in making judgements about questions of life and death - whether as scientists, doctors, patients, relatives or loved ones - these judgements are made against the background of their relationships with human beings and with other animals. These relationships are already in place as the ground from which any moral or ethical system grows. Just as a craftsman's ability to make fine judgements depends on long experience of working with the materials, so the sensitivity of individuals to the needs of others and their capacity to respond to them depends on the historical unfolding of their social relationships, both with human beings and with other animals. Thus, a sense of what may reasonably be done to human beings and to other animals necessarily depends on the sensitivity developed through these relationships.

1.28 In considering the ethical issues raised by xenotransplantation, the Working Party recognised that the capacity to make ethical or moral judgements depends on this sensitivity and that any judgements which had no basis in such experience would carry little practical or motivational force. An attempt has been made to identify principles that will have such a basis but which, at the same time, reflect a critical appraisal of present practice and possible innovation.

Basic assumptions

1.29 This report is based on two assumptions of pluralism. The first is a recognition that it is unrealistic to expect complete consensus across society on the issues addressed in the report. The aim of the report is to seek as much common ethical ground as possible. But it is important to recognise and acknowledge differences of opinion. This will help to inform future debate, to try and ensure that, whichever direction society chooses to take, its decision will be based on principles that can be justified as reasonable to most of its members, and to take account of the views of those who dissent from the majority decision.

1.30 The second assumption is that no single ethical framework can capture all the reasonable perspectives that may be taken on the issues raised by xenotransplantation. The report does not, then, present a particular ethical theory and its application to all the various questions that arise. This would be bound to leave out reasons and values which would not be captured by the theory. Instead, the Working Party attempted to take into account all the salient considerations, to give them whatever weight seemed reasonable, and then to make judgements where appropriate.

Method of working

1.31 The Working Party met 11 times between February 1995 and January 1996. The inquiry was announced in the press in April 1995 and submissions were invited from interested parties. Annex A describes the consultation process in more detail. Written submissions were invited from a wide range of groups and individuals thought to have a possible interest in the issues raised by xenotransplantation. Copies of the consultation letters and information pack are presented in Annex B and those contacted are listed in Annex C. Annex D lists those from whom submissions were received. The Working Party members are grateful to all those who responded.

1.32 The Working Party recognises that the submissions received could not be taken as representative of public opinion as a whole. Their value lay in indicating the range of views on xenotransplantation. Almost all the issues discussed in the report were raised in some form in the submissions and the Working Party has drawn considerably on the thinking set out in them. From the submissions, three main points emerged:

- where responses indicated an overall stance, many were in favour of the further development of xenografts. Most were cautious in this, weighing perceived advantages and disadvantages and specifying the need for a number of safeguards. Views here ranged from those who felt that the present legislation, guidance and codes of practice adequately accommodated developments in this area, to those who wished to see a broadened and continuing development of new regulatory mechanisms;
- a number of respondents expressed the firm view that in no case should xenotransplantation proceed because of their principled objections to the use of animals. In some cases they derived from particular religious convictions. On the whole, the case against xenografts was argued in carefully documented detail: critics were aware of and cited the latest research, and their arguments touched on most or all of the areas of concern that are discussed in the report;
- the weight of comment, regardless of the views expressed, centred on the use of animals.

Use has been made of quotations, selected from the submissions received, throughout the report.

The language used in the report

1.33 The terms **xenotransplantation** and **xenografting** are used interchangeably. The term **organs and tissue** has been used when referring to the xenotransplantation of animal organs, tissue and cells. Where appropriate, organs, tissue and cells are referred to specifically. The term **animals** should be taken to mean **non-human animals**. The Working Party accepts that a limitation of this convention is its suggestion that human beings are separate from other animals, but felt that it could be justified in terms of brevity and clarity. Similarly, the term **primates** should be taken to mean **non-human primates**. The term **source animal**, rather than **donor animal**, has been used in recognition of the fact that an animal has no choice in whether its organs or tissue are removed for human use. To avoid confusion, the term **cost** has been reserved for discussion about the financial implications of xenotransplantation. The term **harm** refers to possible disadvantages either for human beings or for other animals. There is a glossary, defining technical terms, in Annex E.

Chapter 2

Alternatives to xenotransplantation

2.1 The starting point of this enquiry was the widening gap between the demand for, and the supply of, human organs and tissue for transplantation. Xenografts are only one way of closing that gap. In view of the scientific and ethical questions to which xenotransplantation gives rise, it is important to examine other ways of meeting the demand for organs for transplantation. Three approaches will be discussed in this chapter. First, reducing the demand for transplants by promoting health and reducing disease. Second, implementing measures to increase the supply of human organs and, third, developing artificial organs and tissue.

Preventive health measures

2.2 One possible way of bridging the gap between supply and demand is to reduce the demand for human organs and tissue by introducing public health measures to prevent the conditions that currently require treatment by transplantation. For example, the major causes of liver failure in the UK are alcoholism, infection with hepatitis viruses and drug intoxication. In this context, public health measures and policies to encourage healthier lifestyles and to achieve environmental improvements are important. The UK Government published **The Health of the Nation** in 1991, in order to highlight how changes in lifestyle and environmental improvements might contribute to a reduction in the incidence of major diseases.[1] The British Union for the Abolition of Vivisection wrote in their submission: "*Concentrating on improving health and preventing disease, rather than on cures or treatments to repair the damage once it has occurred, is a vastly more sustainable approach.*"

2.3 There are formidable obstacles in the way of measures to improve health and prevent disease. It is often difficult to establish a precise relationship between a lifestyle or environmental factor and a particular disease. Whilst the relationship between excess alcohol consumption and cirrhosis of the liver is clear, the situation is more complicated for most other conditions for which transplants may be required; for example, a high blood cholesterol concentration is one risk factor in coronary heart disease, but there are many others, not least genetic influences and perhaps also environmental factors encountered in fetal life. Cholesterol levels taken in isolation are therefore poor predictors of the likelihood of coronary disease in any one

1 **The Health of the Nation** (1991) London, HMSO Cm 1523.

individual.[2] In addition, devising policies that are effective in changing attitudes and lifestyles is extremely difficult. A study examining different methods of giving dietary advice, for example, found that whether advice was given by a dietician, a practice nurse, or presented in a leaflet, it resulted in only a small reduction in cholesterol levels compared to what might be expected, suggesting that behaviour is difficult to modify.[3] Moreover, many of the diseases currently treated by transplantation are not amenable to preventive approaches and are unlikely to become so in the near future, if at all. These include all the common causes of kidney failure and the cardiomyopathies which afflict young people. Sufferers from cystic fibrosis, an inherited disease, are unlikely to live beyond the third decade without a lung or heart-lung transplant. Finally, any gains made as a result of preventive measures to reduce disease are likely to be long-term ones. In the meantime, the demand for transplantation remains pressing.

Increasing the supply of human organs

2.4 Two recent reports have examined the factors influencing the supply of human organs, and possible ways in which the supply could be increased.[4, 5] The factors affecting human organ donation are many and complicated. Establishing that a particular policy on organ donation does indeed affect the rate of donation is difficult, and many of the factors affecting supply may be either beyond the control of specific policy measures or desirable in their own right. For example, the low rate of organ donation in the UK, compared to some other countries, is due in part to the decline in deaths from road accidents and from brain haemorrhages. Countries with a low population density may have more difficulty collecting and transporting organs and coordinating their transplantation into recipients, though this is not a factor in the UK.

2.5 The level of provision of intensive care units, from which most organ donors come, and of transplant centres also affects transplantation rates. The number of intensive care beds is lower in the UK than in other European countries and there is increasing evidence of a need to expand provision and staffing. Transplant units also suffer from a shortage of surgical staff and transplant coordinators. Increased provision on both fronts would be expected to increase transplantation rates. The National Kidney Federation believes "*there is considerable room for improvement in*

2 Cholesterol: Screening and Treatment. **Effective Health Care**, June 1993, N° 6.

3 Neil H A W *et al.* Randomised trial of lipid lowering dietary advice in general practice: the effects on serum lipids, lipoproteins, and antioxidants. (1995) **British Medical Journal**, 310:569-74.

4 New B *et al.* (1994) **A Question of Give and Take: Improving the supply of donor organs for transplantation.** King's Fund Institute Research Report 18.

5 **Report of the British Transplantation Society Working Party on Organ Donation.** (1995) British Transplantation Society.

medical/nursing training in organ donation. In a study by the Federation in 1991, only 1.5 per cent of undergraduates and 4 per cent of postgraduates described their training in recognition of potential donors as 'good'."[6] Again, improved training would be expected to increase transplantation rates. Spain, which has a well-developed network of transplant coordinators, has seen a steady increase in transplantation rates.[7]

2.6 Efforts could also be made to increase the use of organs from donors whose hearts are no longer beating. Recent studies have suggested that transplantation of kidneys from such donors can be almost as successful as transplantation using heart-beating donors,[8, 9] although another study has questioned this view.[10] Another source of kidneys (and, to a lesser extent, livers) is live donors. In Norway, the high kidney transplant rate is due to the high number of live donors giving kidneys, and recent reports have recommended that kidney donation by live donors should be encouraged in the UK.[11, 12]

2.7 Opinion polls consistently show that, while 70 per cent of UK citizens are in favour of donating their organs after their death, willingness to register as an organ donor is fairly resistant to publicity campaigns, and only about 25 per cent of the population carry organ donor cards.[11] The cards are valuable in that they give a clear indication of the donor's intention to relatives. This is important, since 30 per cent of relatives refuse permission for removal of organs from a potential donor. In an attempt to increase registration, in 1994, the Department of Health introduced a national, computer-based register of potential organ donors.[13] It is too early to determine the effectiveness of this initiative, but, however effective, it is unlikely that it can meet the existing demand for human organs, much less cope with any expansion in that demand.

2.8 One possibility would be to change the law so as to remove the right of relatives to withhold consent to the removal of organs from someone who before dying expressed a wish to donate. A more radical change would be to operate a system of presumed consent in which people who did not wish to have their organs removed would sign a dissent register. Such changes are controversial. Some argue that, given

---

6 Submission to the Working Party.

7 Matesantz R and Miranda B (1995) Letter to **Lancet**, 346:53.

8 Wijnen R M H *et al.* (1995) Outcome of transplantation of non-heart-beating donor kidneys. **Lancet**, 345:1067-70.

9 Andrews P A *et al.* (1995) Letter to **Lancet**, 346:53.

10 Chang R W S (1995) Letter to **Lancet**, 346:322.

11 New B *et al.* (1994) **A Question of Give and Take: Improving the supply of donor organs for transplantation.** King's Fund Institute Research Report 18.

12 **Report of the British Transplantation Society Working Party on Organ Donation.** (1995) British Transplantation Society.

13 For information about the NHS Organ Donor Register, freephone 0800 555777.

the sensitivity of potential organ donors to adverse publicity, more contentious measures to obtain human organs might backfire. Advocates of such changes argue that such legal frameworks have been successful in increasing the supply of human organs in Belgium and Singapore. Yet, establishing that specific policy changes have led to increased transplantation is not easy. In Belgium, for example, an important factor may have been the simultaneous improvement in transplant coordination.

2.9 Another procedure for increasing the supply of human organs is elective ventilation. Elective ventilation involves placing a patient for whom death is inevitable on a ventilator in order to maintain their organs in a suitable state for transplantation. This procedure was used with eight patients in Exeter, between 1988 and 1990.[14] Elective ventilation is contrary to the principle that treatment should be in the best interests of an incapacitated patient, however, and the Department of Health has issued guidance that it is unlawful.[15] This conclusion was supported in a recent report of the Law Commission.[16] A number of bodies, including the British Medical Association[17] and the British Transplantation Society,[18] have concluded that elective ventilation would not be unethical, however, and have recommended that the law should be changed to make it legal. Thus, the issue remains controversial.

2.10 Since 1990 the number of human organ donors has levelled out at about 950 a year.[19] Increased provision of intensive care and transplant facilities, and increased use of donors whose hearts are no longer beating and live donors would go some way to improving transplantation rates. Other measures, such as changing the consent law or introducing elective ventilation, are more controversial and would be regarded by some as unacceptable. Even if all human cadaveric organs were somehow made available for transplant, the supply would still not meet the potential demand.[20] So it is necessary to consider how far the use of artificial organs and tissue may provide an alternative to human organ transplantation.

---

14 Feest T G *et al.* (1990) Protocol for increasing organ donation after cerebrovascular deaths in a district general hospital. **Lancet**, 335:1133-5.

15 Acute Services Policy Unit (1994) **Identification of potential donors of organs for transplantation.** London: Department of Health (HSG(94)1). The situation has been criticised as being unclear due to the existence of another, previously issued, code of practice (Departments of Health of Great Britain and Northern Ireland (1983) **Cadaveric organs for transplantation: a code of practice including the diagnosis of brain death.** London: HMSO). The guidance in this code of practice is ambiguous (Francis R (1995) A legal comment. Letter to **British Medical Journal,** 310:718).

16 Law Commission Report No 231 (1995) **Mental Incapacity.** London: HMSO. pp 94-5.

17 BMA's Ethics, Science and Information Division (1993) **Medical Ethics Today: its practice and philosophy.** BMJ Publishing Group.

18 **Report of the British Transplantation Society Working Party on Organ Donation.** (1995) British Transplantation Society.

19 Information supplied by United Kingdom Transplant Support Service Authority.

20 Caplan A (1992) Is xenografting morally wrong? **Transplantation Proceedings,** 24:722-7, quoted in Tania Woods' submission to the Working Party.

Artificial organs and tissue

2.11 Artificial body parts, from glass eyes to wooden legs, have been used for centuries and offer a possible means of addressing the shortage of organs and tissue for transplantation. Technological advances and modern materials have increased the range and sophistication of artificial implants, but many difficulties remain in replicating the complicated functions of certain human organs. Artificial implants currently under development range from totally mechanical devices to organs consisting of a combination of artificial materials and human cells. The rest of this chapter describes the latest developments in producing artificial organs and indicates where they may become a viable alternative to xenotransplantation.

2.12 The human body is a demanding and hostile environment for artificial tissue and organ replacements: blood has a tendency to clot, it is in constant motion and can be corrosive; tissues may need to bend or stretch and can be subject to sudden shocks; organs may need to adjust their function and output according to the changing demands of the body. The human immune system has evolved to reject substances it recognises as foreign, causing inflammation and blood clots. In addition, artificial devices are susceptible to infectious organisms: even organisms which are not normally dangerous can become deadly when they colonise a foreign object implanted inside the body. Faced by such difficulties, it is perhaps not surprising that most devices currently in use perform fairly basic mechanical or cosmetic functions, and are often located where the blood supply is limited. However, researchers are attempting to develop artificial organs capable of carrying out more sophisticated functions in more difficult environments.

Kidneys

2.13 The longest established procedure for replacing the function of a failing organ with an alternative is dialysis of body fluids in patients with kidney failure. A synthetic membrane, or the peritoneum, is used as a dialysing medium across which the blood can be freed of toxic waste products normally excreted by the kidneys. Patients spend several sessions a week having dialysis, and can live relatively normal lives between treatments, which is not the case when most other organs fail. There has been little research into developing implantable artificial kidneys because patients can be successfully kept alive by dialysis while awaiting transplantation. For many patients, however, dialysis is far from ideal, because it requires lengthy sessions of treatment, restrictions in diet and cannot prevent a general decrease in overall health. As the length of the waiting list for kidney transplants testifies, dialysis does not offer a complete solution to the shortage of kidneys for transplantation.

Heart

2.14 Of all implantable mechanical organs, most progress has been made with artificial heart devices.[21] This is because the operation of the heart is fairly simple (it is basically a pump) and, unlike many other organs, it performs only limited biochemical or metabolic functions. Two types of artificial hearts are being developed: ventricular assist devices and total artificial hearts.

2.15 Ventricular assist devices (VAD) are at a more advanced stage of development than totally artificial hearts. Ventricular assist devices support but do not replace the heart, which remains in place and continues to perform some functions. Left ventricular assist devices (LVADs) are the most common type and help the left ventricle of the heart pump blood around the body. Since 80 per cent of the work of the heart is done by the left ventricle, LVADs are the most important type of artificial heart. Right ventricular assist devices (RVADs) help pump blood to the lungs for oxygenation, and can be used in conjunction with LVADs.

2.16 Most LVADs are implanted in the abdomen. A small lead through the skin attaches the LVAD to batteries, which are carried in a pack on a belt. The LVAD can keep time with the natural heartbeat and a computer adjusts the pumping action to cope with changes in activity. Patients have lived with the aid of an LVAD for up to two years. Currently, LVADs are used on a short-term basis, to keep a patient alive until a human organ is available. Supported by an LVAD, the heart can rest and, in some cases may recover sufficiently to allow the device to be removed after which the patient's condition can be managed with drugs. Thus, LVADs could in principle be used as an early form of treatment for heart disease before the condition becomes life-threatening. Also being developed are intra-ventricular artificial hearts which are so small they can be implanted into the heart itself. These devices have the potential to be used on a long-term basis as an alternative to human organ transplantation.

2.17 Total artificial hearts are designed to carry out all of the main functions of the heart. Several designs have been tried, but all follow the same basic principles, in which chambers pump blood to the lungs for oxygenation and then around the rest of the body. In 1982, a patient was kept alive for 112 days with a total artificial heart. Development continues and the devices have potential for short-term use in patients suffering from biventricular heart failure who are waiting for a human organ.

2.18 Artificial hearts may eventually provide an alternative for patients waiting for a human organ and they do not require the use of immunosuppressive drugs. But there are various problems to be overcome with the use of artificial hearts:

21 Reviewed in Westaby S (1996) The need for artificial hearts. **British Heart Journal,** in press.

- since blood tends to react with nearly every artificial substance, clots can form inside the devices and may cause strokes if they dislodge and travel through the circulation to the brain. Researchers are attempting to produce materials that reduce the tendency of blood to clot. One approach is to use the patient's own endothelial cells to line the surfaces of the device that are in contact with blood. In the meantime, patients are treated with anticoagulant drugs to reduce the tendency of the blood to clot;

- artificial hearts tend to damage blood cells, causing anaemia and sometimes liver and kidney problems. Such damage is reduced by designing devices which allow a less turbulent blood flow;

- the power supplies are bulky and inconvenient, and need frequent recharging; often the person must be connected to a recharging unit at night. Because of their size, and the heat they generate, the power units cannot be implanted. The lead connecting the heart to a power supply outside the body can cause problems with infections;

- the devices are very expensive, costing about £30,000 each.

Thus, for the foreseeable future at least, mechanical hearts are unlikely to satisfy the demand for heart transplants.

Lungs

2.19 The first artificial lung capable of oxygenating blood and eliminating carbon dioxide was developed in the 1950s.[22] These devices were located outside the body and were used for periods of up to five hours to support patients during heart surgery when it was necessary to bypass the function of the heart and lungs. In 1992, a patient survived for 45 days with the aid of extracorporeal membrane oxygenation in which blood is removed from the body, oxygenated and returned to the body. This technique is now in clinical use for treating lung failure, especially in infants, but it remains a short-term measure.

2.20 Trials of implantable oxygenating devices are now in progress. The intravascular oxygenator is a miniature membrane lung which can be placed inside the body. The heart pumps blood through the device (unlike external devices which require external pumps) and gas is exchanged through microporous polypropylene fibres. The efficiency of the gas exchange depends greatly upon the surface area of the membrane, and therefore on the size of the devices. Thus, small implantable devices are not as efficient as external artificial lungs.

---

22 Goldsmith M (1993) After two decades Penn State researchers may be near perfecting replacement hearts and lungs. **Journal of the American Medical Association**, 269:966-973.

2.21 Infection is a major problem with artificial lungs, since they are in constant contact with the atmosphere and do not have the natural protection mechanisms found in human lungs. Blood clotting is another problem that must be overcome before artificial lung implants become a realistic option.

Bioengineered organ and tissue replacements

2.22 As indicated above, reproducing the complicated functions of the body in a purely mechanical way is extremely difficult. This has led to the development of artificial organs incorporating living cells, tissues or organs which can perform some of the functions of the tissue or organ that needs replacing.

Liver

2.23 The liver performs a wide range of important functions including the processing of the products of digestion, the control of the metabolism of proteins and carbohydrates, the manufacture of essential proteins such as blood clotting factors, the removal of toxic substances absorbed from the gut, the excretion of the breakdown products of red blood cells and the secretion of bile. It is impossible at present to begin to replicate all of these complicated functions by wholly artificial means, so research has focused instead upon bioengineered livers. The intention is to use them on a short-term basis to keep patients suffering from liver failure alive while they wait for a transplant or to give their own liver a chance to regenerate. At the simplest level, the patient's blood is passed through an animal liver: at best this can keep patients alive for a very short time.[23]

2.24 Implantable artificial livers are a long way off, but clinical trials are under way for artificial livers which function outside the body. One such device is the extracorporeal liver assist device, which has been used successfully in small numbers of patients.[24] The device filters blood through thousands of tiny porous tubes. Human liver cells are packed around the tubes to process the passing blood and to get rid of waste. The liver cells are immortalised (they have the ability to keep reproducing) and can be grown in the laboratory. It is important that the liver cells do not enter the blood, as there is a chance that if they passed into the body and became established in an organ or tissue, they might develop into tumours.

23 Chari R *et al.* (1994) Brief report: Treatment of hepatic failure with *ex vivo* pig-liver perfusion followed by liver transplantation. **New England Journal of Medicine,** 331:234-7.

24 McNair A N B *et al.* (1995) Recent advances : hepatology. **British Medical Journal,** 311:1351-5.

2.25 Other devices contain pig liver cells. The person's blood is separated before treatment, with the cells being removed and only plasma entering the device. Eliminating the cells reduces the risk of blood clot formation, but the lack of red blood cells means that the liver cells in the machine suffer from a lack of oxygen. Alternative methods of supplying the liver cells with oxygen have been tried, but so far the cells have died within eight hours or so.

2.26 A different approach is to try and produce a true replacement liver grown in the laboratory.[25] An artificial scaffolding rather like a sponge is produced, made either from biodegradable or from tough and inert material. Blood vessels and liver cells are encouraged to grow onto the scaffolding. If successful, organs made in this way could then be used for transplantation. All these methods of liver replacement, however, are far from becoming routine clinical procedures.

Pancreatic islet cells

2.27 Like the liver, the pancreas performs complicated biochemical functions which are difficult to replicate by artificial means. Efforts have been made to improve the success of transplantation of living islets of Langerhans, the pancreatic cells that produce insulin.[26] This would be used to treat patients suffering from diabetes. The islet cells are encapsulated in a porous membrane that does not cause an immune response. Blood passes through the membrane, and the trapped pancreatic cells produce insulin and help regulate the level of blood sugar. Since the islet cells remain separate from the blood, and from the cells of the recipient's immune system, there is no immune response to the transplant. This suggests that the pancreatic cells could be supplied by non-compatible human donors or by other animals.

Bones and joints

2.28 Techniques for repairing bones and joints using artificial materials are well established, and have become more successful with improvements in the materials used. These must be tough, lightweight, corrosion resistant and they must not cause an immune response. Stainless steel, used in hip replacements, and bone cements, however, shield the surrounding bone from stress and lead to wasting of the natural material. Thus, there is considerable interest in developing bioengineered bone in

25 Miller S K (1992) Cells and sponge support failing liver. **New Scientist,** 1 August 1992, p 20.

26 Soon-Shiong P *et al.* (1994) Insulin independence in a type 1 diabetic patient after encapsulated islet transplantation. **Lancet,** 343:950-1.

which an artificial framework or matrix is transplanted into the body.[27] This encourages surrounding cells to enter the matrix and leads to new bone growth. Alternatively, cells can be seeded onto the matrix before transplantation. Since the patient's own bone marrow cells can be used, rejection is not a problem.

2.29 The shortage of bone for transplantation is not as acute as the shortage of organs and some other tissue. This is partly because autografting, in which bone from one part of the body is used to repair bone in another part of the patient's body, is a relatively common technique. Human bone can also be stored for long periods which makes it easier to maintain a supply for transplantation. Nevertheless, there is some interest in xenotransplantation and limited use has already been made of transplant material derived from cow bone.[28]

Skin

2.30 Rapid advances have been made recently in producing skin grown from human cells.[29] This can be used to treat burns and ulcers. Cells from one of the skin's layers, the dermis, are grown on a biodegradable matrix to produce a sheet of dermis cells. After transplantation of a dermis layer to cover a wound, the patient's own outer layer of skin (the epidermis) grows over the transplanted dermis. Another method takes skin from corpses and treats it to remove the cells, leaving a weave of protein fibres, including collagen. When this protein matrix is grafted onto a wound, it is quickly colonised by the recipient's own skin cells and blood vessels. Because the transplanted matrix does not contain cells, it does not provoke an immune response and is tolerated well by recipients.

2.31 Like bone, a number of strategies are available to replace skin. Autografting, in which skin from one part of the body is grafted elsewhere is possible. Skin can be stored for up to three years, making its collection from corpses, and after operations such as cosmetic surgery, possible. Xenotransplantation of pig skin to treat burns patients has been used in the past but is no longer common. Should the development of transgenic pigs allow transplantation of pig organs and tissue without a strong immune response, then interest in xenotransplantation of pig skin may revive. Recent developments have involved the growth of skin cells on three-dimensional supports.[29] This raises the possibility of replacing complicated three-dimensional structures such as the ear. Ultimately it is hoped that these techniques will permit the production of bioengineered heart valves and even organs.

---

27 Crane G M *et al.* (1995) Bone tissue engineering. **Nature Medicine,** 1:1322-4.

28 Poumarat G and Squire P (1993) Comparison of mechanical properties of human, bovine bone and a new processed bone xenograft. **Biomaterials,** 14:337-40.

29 Dickman S and Strobel G (1995) Life in the tissue factory. **New Scientist,** 11 March 1995, pp 32-7.

Conclusion

2.32 There are problems in closing the gap between the demand for transplantation and the supply of donor organs. Preventive measures may go some way towards meeting the demand but are necessarily long-term and of uncertain effectiveness. Increasing the supply of organs from human donors is difficult and, in some cases, not without ethical complications. Mechanical and bioengineered organ replacements, while offering future promise, remain problematical for the time being. This means that attention has turned to the use of animal organs as one potential method of satisfying the demand for transplantation. The next chapter assesses the progress that has been made towards developing successful xenotransplantation.

Chapter 3

Xenotransplantation : progress and prospects

3.1 A key question raised by xenotransplantation is whether or not the technique will work. In this chapter the scientific background to xenotransplantation is set out to provide a basis for the discussion of the ethical issues that follows in subsequent chapters.

3.2 Table 3.1 gives examples of the main xenotransplantation procedures involving human recipients that have occurred to date. A wide range of procedures has been used. Some of them are now routine, such as the use of pig heart valves to replace the patient's own defective valves. Far more ambitious and, to date, unsuccessful are attempts to replace defective human organs, such as the heart, liver or kidneys, with transplanted animal organs. There are two major practical problems that have to be faced.

3.3 First, there is the problem of organ rejection. When a human organ is transplanted from one individual into another, the recipient's immune system attacks the organ because it is seen as foreign (the sole exception is transplantation between identical twins). If the immune response is extreme, the organ will be rejected and the transplant will fail. This is why human donor organs are matched with those of transplant patients as closely as possible. Even with closely matched organs, however, immunosuppressive drugs have to be used to subdue the response of the patient's immune system to the transplanted organ.

3.4 Organ rejection becomes much more of a problem with xenografting, because of the greater difference between human and animal tissues. The more distantly related, in a biological sense, the human recipient and the source animal, the stronger the immune reaction. For this reason, attempts have been made in the US to use organs from primates, such as baboons, for xenotransplantation. Biologically speaking, primates are closely related to human beings so that problems of organ rejection may not be much more severe than those seen with human transplants. As discussed in Chapter 4, however, ethical concerns are raised by the use of primates for xenotransplantation. So efforts have been made to develop animals other than primates for use in xenografting. Attention has focused in particular on the pig for several reasons. Pig organs are comparable in size and, to a lesser degree, physiology to those of human beings, and they reproduce quickly and produce large numbers of offspring. The use of pigs as a domestic animal that is farmed and eaten is long established and many would have fewer concerns about their use for xenotransplantation as compared with the use of primates (discussed further in Chapter 4).

3.5 Pigs, however, are less closely related to human beings than primates. The human immune response to pig organs is rapid and severe, resulting in complete destruction of the transplanted organ. This is called **hyperacute rejection.**[1] Hyperacute rejection is so extreme that it cannot be controlled with immunosuppressive drugs. The success of pig heart valve transplantation lies in the fact that they can be treated with a preservative (glutaraldehyde) that reduces the strength of the immune response they induce.[2] This cannot be done with organs because they must be fully viable when they are transplanted. Instead, one promising approach for preventing organ rejection involves modifying the pig organs so that they do not cause such a strong immune response when transplanted into human beings. This is done by altering the genetic make-up of the pig by introducing human genetic material, producing **transgenic** pigs.[3] There is evidence from experiments with animal recipients that the immune response is reduced when transgenic pig organ or tissue is transplanted.

3.6 The second problem raised by xenotransplantation is whether an animal organ will be able to perform the functions that a healthy human organ does. The heart is a relatively simple mechanical pump, so an animal heart, in principle, should be able to perform the same function. It is clearly important, however, that the animal organs are about same size as human ones. Other organs, notably the liver, have complicated biochemical functions that may differ between species. Proteins produced by an animal liver may be functionally incompatible with those of a human recipient. It is simply not known whether an animal liver will support human life. Finally, differences in life span must be considered. The natural life span of the pig is about 20 years.[4] Would a transplanted pig organ age more rapidly than the human recipient? If so, this might lead to the need for successive transplants throughout the lifetime of the recipient.

3.7 The next sections describe the scope of the report and provide some background about the immune response and organ rejection. Experience with the use of primates for xenotransplantation is described. Then, the problem of reducing the immune response to xenografted pig organs is discussed, and the different approaches for overcoming hyperacute rejection are described.

---

1 Reviewed in Rowe P M (January 1996) Xenotransplantation: from animal facility to the clinic? **Molecular Medicine Today**, pp 10-15, and Fabre J W (1995) Nudging xenotransplantation towards humans. **Nature Medicine**, 1:403-4.

2 Marks C and Marks P (1993) **Fundamentals of cardiac surgery.** London: Chapman & Hall Medical, pp 105-9.

3 Cozzi E and White D J G (1995) The generation of transgenic pigs as potential organ donors for humans. **Nature Medicine,** 1:964-6.

4 Holliday R (1995) Letter to **Nature,** 378:434.

Table 3.1 Examples of the major xenotransplantation procedures involving human recipients that have occurred to date

Primates All operations took place in the US.	
1964	Six patients received chimpanzee kidneys. Most died within days. One survived nine months.[5]
1964	Six patients received baboon kidneys. All died within two months.[6]
1984	Baby Fae received a baboon heart. She survived 20 days.[7]
1992	Patient received a baboon liver and survived 70 days.[8]
1993	Patient received a baboon liver and survived 26 days.[9]
1995	AIDS patient received a baboon bone marrow transplant in December. He left hospital in January 1996, at which point it was not known whether the transplant had been successful.[10, 11]
Other animals	
1964	The first UK pig heart valve transplant took place. Now a routine operation.[12]
1968	Patient received sheep heart and died instantly.[13]
1992	Patient received pig heart and survived less than 24 hours.[13]
1994	Ten Swedish diabetic patients received pig fetal islet cells. In four patients, the pig cells survived for up to 14 months. Insulin produced at extremely low levels.[14, 15]
1995	Four Parkinson's patients received pig fetal neural tissue in the US.[16]

5 Reemtsma K B *et al.* (1964) Renal heterotransplantation in man. **Annals of Surgery,** 160:384.

6 Starzl T E *et al.* (1964) Renal heterotransplantation from baboon to man: experience with 6 cases. **Transplantation,** 2:752-76.

7 Bailey L L *et al.* (1985) Baboon-to-human cardiac xenotransplantation in a neonate. **Journal of the American Medical Association,** 254:3321-9.

8 Starzl T E *et al.* (1993) Baboon-to-human liver transplantation. **Lancet,** 341:65-71.

9 Starzl T E *et al.* (1994) Clinical xenotransplantation. **Xenotransplant,** 1:3-7.

10 AIDS patient given baboon bone marrow (1995) **Nature,** 378:756.

11 Baboon man leaves hospital (1996) **New Scientist,** 13 January 1996, p 6.

12 Marks C and Marks P (1993) **Fundamentals of cardiac surgery.** London: Chapman & Hall Medical, pp 105-9.

13 Mentioned in Dunning J, White D and Wallwork J (1994) The rationale for xenotransplantation as a solution to the donor organ shortage. **Pathologie Biologie,** 42:231-5.

14 Groth C G *et al.* (1994) Transplantation of porcine fetal pancreas to diabetic patients. **Lancet,** 344:1402-4.

15 Nowak R (1994) Pig transplants offer hope in diabetes. **Science,** 266:1323.

16 Parkinson's pig cure. **The Times,** 15 December 1995.

Definition and scope of xenotransplantation

3.8 **Transplantation** involves the removal of cells, tissue or organs from one organism and their implantation into another organism. **Xenotransplantation** or **xenografting** refers to transplantation between different species. The scope of this report is restricted to the relatively new developments in xenotransplantation of **organs, tissue or cells**. The transfer of **molecules** between species, as in the use of pig insulin for treating human diabetics, is not normally thought of as xenotransplantation, and lies outside the scope of this report. If xenotransplantation involving organs, tissue and cells is found to be ethically acceptable, however, then it is unlikely that there will be objections to the transfer of molecules from one species to another. Conversely, even if it is considered ethically acceptable to use animals to provide molecules for human benefit, there may well be objections to the use of their organs, tissue or cells. The transfer of **genetic material** between species is also not usually thought of as xenotransplantation. It is discussed in this report in the context of the production of transgenic animals for xenografting (paragraphs 4.45 - 4.54 and 5.9 - 5.17).

The immune response

3.9 The function of the immune system is to protect the body from disease. The immune response is divided into two: the **antibody response** and the **cell-mediated response.** Both responses depend on white blood cells, the main component of the immune system.[17]

3.10 Any infectious organisms entering the body, such as bacteria or viruses, have molecules called **antigens** on their surface. These antigens are recognised as foreign by the immune system and an immune response is mounted to protect the body from infection. Unfortunately, an immune response is also induced by transplantation. This is because organs and tissues also have antigens on their surface. Some of these antigens vary between individuals. When an organ is transplanted from a human donor into a patient, the patient's immune system recognises the antigens on the transplanted organ as different, or foreign, and an immune response is triggered. If the immune response is very strong, the transplanted organ or tissue may be rejected. Whether the immune response occurs in response to infectious organisms or to a transplant, the basic elements are as described below.

3.11 An important element of the immune response is due to **antibodies**. Antibodies are produced by a type of white blood cell, called B-cells. Antibodies are molecules that circulate in the blood and stick to foreign antigens. This may inactivate the foreign organisms or the cells of the transplant directly, or it may enable other white blood

17 Roitt I (1994) **Essential Immunology** Eighth Edition. Oxford: Blackwell Scientific Publications.

cells to destroy them. One important consequence of antibodies sticking to antigens is the activation of a complicated reaction called the **complement** reaction.

3.12 Complement is a system of more than twenty different blood proteins. When antibodies stick to antigens, a reaction is triggered, with one complement protein activating the next, and so on. Ultimately, the complement proteins at the end of the chain attack the foreign organisms or the cells of a transplanted organ, punching holes in them and thus destroying them.

3.13 Clearly, it is important that the complement proteins do not attack the body's own cells. In order to prevent this, human cells have on their surface **complement regulating proteins** that prevent the activation of complement proteins. The most important of these molecules are called DAF, CD59 and MCP.[18]

3.14 The cell-mediated immune response depends on another class of white blood cell, called T-cells. Killer T-cells directly attack cells bearing foreign antigens, including the cells of transplanted organs, ultimately killing them. For the transplantation of human organs, the cell-mediated response of the T-cells is more important for organ rejection than the antibody response.

Preventing organ rejection

3.15 While the immune response is beneficial when directed towards foreign organisms, it is clearly undesirable when directed towards a transplanted organ. Such is the strength of the human immune response that transplantation of human organs between unrelated individuals was a dangerous and experimental procedure until the 1970s. There are two main approaches for reducing the immune response and preventing organ rejection.

3.16 First, the antigens on the transplanted organ are matched with the recipient's antigens as closely as possible in order to reduce the immune response. There are many different antigens, and each one varies widely between individuals. This means that it is almost impossible to get a perfect tissue match between individuals (except between identical twins).

3.17 Second, the patient's immune system can be suppressed with immunosuppressive drugs to help prevent rejection of mismatched transplants. The major drawback of immunosuppression is that it interferes with the operation of the immune system as a whole. This means that the patient has increased susceptibility to infections and to certain types of cancer. Immunosuppressive drugs work in different ways. Some,

18 DAF stands for 'decay accelerating factor' and MCP for 'membrane co-factor protein'. CD59 is a member of a group of cell surface molecules called CD antigens.

such as cyclosporin A, inhibit T-cell activity. Other drugs, for example azathioprine, reduce the numbers of T-cells. Another drug, cyclophosphamide, inhibits the production of antibodies, and prednisone reduces inflammation.[19]

Xenotransplantation of primate organs and tissue

3.18 The more closely related two species are, the more antigens they will have in common, and the weaker the recipient's immune response will be. Genetically, the higher primates are remarkably similar to human beings: the genetic material of our closest relative, the chimpanzee, differs from that of human beings by just 2 per cent.[20] Accordingly, many antigens are shared, and few differ. Thus, the immune response when a human receives a primate xenograft is broadly similar to the response to a poorly matched human organ.[21] However, very close tissue matching when donor and recipient are from different species is impossible and rejection is therefore correspondingly stronger than that seen with human transplants.

3.19 Xenotransplantation between closely related species, where the immune response is not too extreme, is called **concordant xenografting.** Rejection of concordant xenografts, as of human transplants, is usually because of the action of T-cells. In practice, organs transplanted from concordant species are handled in a broadly similar way to human transplants where donor and recipient tissues are poorly matched. Immunosuppressive drugs are used to prevent rejection of concordant xenografts although so far with less success than for human transplants. With continuing advances in the effectiveness of immunosuppressive drugs, however, it may become possible to control the immune response to concordant xenografts.

3.20 Of the several attempts made in the United States to transplant primate organs into human beings, none has been successful (Table 3.1). In a series of experiments in the 1960s, patients were transplanted with chimpanzee or baboon kidneys. Most of these patients died within days but one recipient of a chimpanzee kidney survived nine months. This is remarkable, given the limitations of the immunosuppressive drugs available at that time. Due to the endangered status of chimpanzees, their use as a source of organs is no longer acceptable (Chapter 4), and attention has turned to the use of baboons. Much interest was raised by the case of Baby Fae, born with a defective heart, who received a transplanted baboon heart in 1984. Baby Fae survived 20 days. More recently, there have been two attempts to transplant a baboon liver into patients suffering from liver failure. One of these recipients survived 26 days, the other 70 days.

19 Roitt I (1994) **Essential Immunology** Eighth Edition. Oxford: Blackwell Scientific Publications, pp 348-50.

20 Diamond J (1993) The Third Chimpanzee, Chapter 8 of Cavalieri P and Singer P, eds. **The Great Ape Project.** London: Fourth Estate.

21 Starzl T E *et al.* (1993) Baboon-to-human liver transplantation. **Lancet**, 341:65-71.

Baboon bone marrow transplants for treating AIDS patients

3.21 Another rather different use has been proposed for baboon xenografts. This stems from the observation that baboons, unlike most other primates, are resistant to infection with the HIV virus that causes AIDS. It has been proposed to transplant baboon bone marrow into patients suffering from the advanced stages of AIDS, in an attempt to restore the function of the immune system. This proposal has been approved by the Food and Drug Administration of the United States.[22] There are, however, several difficulties with the procedure. It is not clear that baboon bone marrow will transplant successfully into human beings. There is a risk that the baboon bone marrow will attack the patient's body in what is called graft versus host disease. Moreover, it is not known whether baboon bone marrow will be able to restore the functions lacking in the patient's immune system. In addition, as described in Chapter 6, there are serious concerns about the risk that xenotransplantation of baboon tissue will enable primate diseases to pass into the human population. Nevertheless, an AIDS patient received a bone marrow xenograft in the US in December 1995.[23]

Will primate organs function properly in human beings?

3.22 One problem in xenotransplantation is caused by the disparity in size of human and primate organs. An adult male baboon, for example, weighs only about 22-30 kg,[24] less than half the average weight of an adult human being, and the organs are correspondingly smaller than human organs. This means that a baboon heart would not be powerful enough to pump blood around the body of an adult human being. There is an acute shortage, however, of very small human organs for transplantation into babies suffering from heart malformations. This has led to the suggestion that primate organs might be transplanted into children as a temporary solution, or bridge, while they wait for a suitable human organ to become available. This suggestion is discussed further in Chapter 7 (paragraphs 7.22 - 7.24). Consideration must also be given to whether primate organs will be able to perform the biochemical and physiological functions required in human beings.

22 Pennisi E (1995) FDA Panel OKs baboon marrow transplant. **Science,** 269:293-4.

23 AIDS patient given baboon bone marrow (1995) **Nature,** 378:756.

24 Whitney R A and Wickings E J (1987) Macaques and other old world simians, Chapter 40 of **The UFAW Handbook on the Care and Management of Laboratory Animals** Sixth Edition. UK: Longman Scientific & Technical.

Xenotransplantation of pig organs and tissue

3.23 The ethical and scientific difficulties in using primate organs and tissue for xenotransplantation have led to interest in using pigs, but the immune response if a pig organ is transplanted into a human being is extremely strong. Xenotransplantation of this type, between distantly related species in which the immune response is rapid and extreme, is called **discordant xenografting.** The immediate effect seen after transplantation of a discordant xenograft is called **hyperacute rejection.** This is a fast, violent reaction in which a discordant xenograft can be destroyed within minutes.

Hyperacute rejection

3.24 Hyperacute rejection occurs because human beings have antibodies in their circulation which recognise antigens on the cells of pigs and all other distantly related species, triggering a rapid immune response.[25] As blood flows through the animal organ, antibodies bind to the antigens on the endothelial cells lining the blood vessels of the organ. The complement system is activated and the xenograft is attacked. Complement proteins also activate the immune system's white blood cells which then attack the xenograft. Within minutes the xenograft is reduced to a black, swollen mass. Unlike solid organs, tissues such as bone marrow do not have major blood vessels passing through them. This means that hyperacute rejection is not such a problem.

3.25 For pig organs, however, preventing hyperacute rejection will be a crucial first step towards successful xenotransplantation. One promising method for achieving this is to modify the pigs genetically so that they carry human complement regulating proteins (DAF, CD59 or MCP) on the surface of their cells.[26, 27] These are the proteins that prevent complement being activated (paragraph 3.13). The idea is that when an organ from a modified pig is transplanted into a human being, the human complement regulating proteins on the cells of the pig organ will inhibit the activation of complement. The method of modification involves introducing the human gene that produces the complement regulating protein into the pig.

25 Reviewed in Rowe P M (January 1996) Xenotransplantation: from animal facility to the clinic? **Molecular Medicine Today,** pp 10-15, and Fabre J W (1995) Nudging xenotransplantation towards humans. **Nature Medicine,** 1:403-4.

26 Cozzi E and White D J G (1995) The generation of transgenic pigs as potential organ donors for humans. **Nature Medicine,** 1:964-6.

27 McCurry K R *et al.* (1995) Human complement regulatory proteins protect swine-to-primate cardiac xenografts from humoral injury. **Nature Medicine,** 1:423-7.

3.26 The process of introducing a gene into an animal is called transgenesis. It has been possible to produce transgenic animals for more than ten years. These are mostly transgenic mice used for research purposes. Transgenic farm animals are now in existence which can produce human proteins for therapeutic purposes. For example, sheep have been transgenically modified to produce a human protein called AAT (α1-antitrypsin) which protects the lungs. Ultimately, this protein will be used to treat people who cannot produce their own AAT and who suffer from emphysema.[28]

3.27 The first step is to induce mature female pigs to produce many eggs by treatment with hormones. The sows are then mated and the fertilised eggs are removed. The human gene is introduced into each egg by use of a very fine glass needle guided by a microscope. A gene transferred in this manner is known as a **transgene**. In a small percentage of animals the transgene will be incorporated into the pig's genetic material and will be expressed in every cell of the body, including the cells of the germline, so that if these animals are subsequently bred, their offspring will also carry the transgene and inherit the modification.

3.28 The treated fertilised eggs or early embryos are implanted into a surrogate mother, which may need to be treated with hormones to accept the implant. When the offspring are born, techniques are used to identify which ones are transgenic, and carry the desired gene. These animals usually have the transgene in only one of a pair of chromosomes (they are heterozygotes). By selective breeding, transgenic animals can be produced in which both chromosomes of a pair have copies of the transgene (homozygotes).

3.29 The UK company Imutran Ltd has produced transgenic pigs that contain the human complement regulating protein, DAF.[29] Hearts from these pigs have been transplanted into ten cynomolgus monkeys. In two of the monkeys the hearts were still beating after 60 days. In comparison, unmodified pig hearts lasted just under an hour after transplantation before they were destroyed by hyperacute rejection.[30] In the US, transgenic pigs containing human CD59 have been produced.[31] Hearts transplanted into baboons lasted up to 30 hours whereas unmodified pig hearts lasted about an hour.

28 Sheep to produce α1-antitrypsin (1992) **British Medical Journal**, 304:527.

29 Cozzi E and White D J G (1995) The generation of transgenic pigs as potential organ donors for humans. **Nature Medicine**, 1:964-6.

30 Thompson C (1995) Humanised pigs hearts boost xenotransplantation. **Lancet**, 346:766.

31 McCurry K R *et al.* (1995) Human complement regulatory proteins protect swine-to-primate cardiac xenografts from humoral injury. **Nature Medicine**, 1:423-7.

3.30 A slightly different approach is to modify pigs so that they no longer have the pig antigens that mark them as different from human beings. The most important pig antigen is the sugar molecule galactosyl α-1,3-galactose (here called α-gal).[32] This is recognised by the human antibodies which trigger hyperacute rejection. One strategy would be to remove the pig gene which produces α-gal so it was no longer present on the pig's cells. Deleting a gene from an animal requires embryonic stem cells which can be grown in the laboratory. This allows the appropriate gene to be deleted from the cells, after which the cells are placed into developing embryos. The resulting offspring will contain some tissue that developed from the embryonic stem cells and which does not contain the gene. Suitable pig embryonic stem cells are not yet available, although this approach has been used successfully in mice.

3.31 Since genes cannot be deleted from pigs at the moment, a different strategy has to be used in order to reduce the levels of α-gal pig antigen. This involves making transgenic pigs containing a human gene which has the effect of reducing the levels of α-gal antigen. The transgenic pigs contain the human α-1,2-fucosyltransferase gene. This gene makes the pigs produce a different antigen and a competition is set up: in producing the new antigen, the pigs produce less of the α-gal antigen that causes hyperacute rejection.[33]

3.32 It would, in principle, be possible to breed animals containing two or more different transgenes. For example, if an animal with the DAF transgene were mated with an animal with the α-1,2-fucosyltransferase transgene, some of the offspring would have both transgenes. The hope would be that the presence of two complement regulating proteins might allow more effective complement inhibition if the organs were transplanted into human beings.

Other methods for reducing hyperacute rejection

3.33 A different approach is to try and make the human recipient tolerant of the xenografted organ or tissue so that an immune response is not induced. There is evidence that if an animal receives a bone marrow transplant from an animal of a different, but closely related, species, the recipient can subsequently receive other transplants from the same source animal without mounting a strong immune response.[34] Attempts to transplant pig bone marrow into primates have not yet been successful. In principle, however, it might prove easier to transplant pig bone marrow than pig organs since, like other tissue, it is not susceptible to hyperacute rejection (paragraph 3.24), although graft versus host disease can be a problem

32 Platt J L and Parker W (1995) Another step towards xenotransplantation. **Nature Medicine,** 1:1248-50.

33 Sandrin M S *et al.* (1995) Enzymatic remodelling of the carbohydrate surface of a xenogenic cell substantially reduces human antibody binding and complement-mediated cytolysis. **Nature Medicine,** 1:1261-7.

34 Sachs D H *et al.* (1995) Tolerance and xenograft survival. **Nature Medicine,** 1:969.

(paragraph 3.21). The eventual aim would be to give people bone marrow transplants from a source animal. Once tolerance was induced, other organs could be transplanted.

3.34 A number of other methods have been used to try and prevent, or reduce, hyperacute rejection.[35] One approach is to remove the antibodies that recognise pig antigens from the blood of the human recipient. In principle this could be done by passing the person's blood through a filter that contains the pig antigen. The antibodies would stick to the antigen in the filter and thus be removed from the blood. This would allow a xenograft to take place. The human recipient would eventually make more antibodies but it is possible that the pig tissue would not be destroyed at that stage. Another approach is to treat the pig organ with fragments of antibody before transplantation which cover up the antigens and stop the body's antibodies sticking to them. Finally, it is possible to try and treat the recipient with substances that inhibit the complement system.[36] Cobra venom factor acts as a complement inhibitor. Alternatively, one of the body's natural complement inhibitors, soluble complement receptor type 1, can be made artificially and used to try and prevent hyperacute rejection. It is not yet clear whether these methods will be useful for clinical xenotransplantation.

Other obstacles to xenotransplantation using pig organs

3.35 Thus, a number of methods for preventing, or reducing, hyperacute rejection are being developed. If hyperacute rejection can indeed be controlled, there will be other elements of the immune system to overcome.[37] Since most discordant xenografts are destroyed by hyperacute rejection, little is known about these other elements but they may have a significant role in organ rejection. First, there is likely to be an additional antibody response, less vigorous than hyperacute rejection and similar to the antibody response seen in human organ transplantation. Second, there will be a cell-mediated response, in which T-cells attack the xenograft. T-cells, however, must interact with the cells they are attacking. Since the cells of a pig xenograft are very different to human cells, the T-cells may not be able to interact with them very effectively and so it is possible that the cell-mediated response to a xenograft may be less severe, in some respects, than the response to a human transplant. Finally, xenografts, like human transplants, may be susceptible to chronic rejection. This slow process happens over months or years, and leads to damage to the blood vessels of the transplant. Even in human organ transplantation, this process is not

35 Reviewed in Rowe P M (January 1996) Xenotransplantation: from animal facility to the clinic? **Molecular Medicine Today**, pp 10-15, and Fabre J W (1995) Nudging xenotransplantation towards humans. **Nature Medicine**, 1:403-4.

36 Ryan U S (1995) Complement inhibitory therapeutics and xenotransplantation. **Nature Medicine,** 1:967-8.

37 Bachs F H *et al.* (1995) Barriers to xenotransplantation. **Nature Medicine,** 1:869-73.

understood. Nevertheless, the UK company Imutran Ltd have announced their intention to start trials transplanting transgenic pig organs into human patients in 1996.[38] Xenotransplantation of pig fetal neural tissue is currently taking place in the US.[39]

Conclusion

3.36 To date, attempts to treat people by xenotransplantation have not been successful. There has been recent progress in overcoming some of the difficulties in preventing xenograft rejection, but many obstacles remain. Despite advances in the effectiveness of immunosuppressive drugs, the levels of immunosuppression required to prevent rejection of primate xenografts leave patients susceptible to lethal infections.[40] The small size of primate organs is also likely to cause problems. Where xenotransplantation of pig organs is concerned, the first problem is to control hyperacute rejection. The most promising approach is the development of transgenic pigs containing human proteins that inhibit the complement reaction to a xenografted organ. Even if hyperacute rejection can be controlled, there will be other immunological barriers to acceptance of the xenograft by the recipient. There may also be biochemical and physiological incompatibilities between pig organs and human beings.

3.37 The current attempts to develop xenotransplantation raise the questions whether the use of animals to provide organs and tissue for transplantation is acceptable and, if so, how their welfare can best be taken into account. These questions are discussed in Chapters 4 and 5.

38 Pig-to-human heart transplant slated to begin in 1996 (1995) **Nature Medicine**, 1:987.

39 Parkinson's pig cure. **The Times**, 15 December 1995.

40 Starzl T *et al.* (1994) Clinical xenotransplantation. **Xenotransplant**, 1:3-7.

Chapter 4

Animal concerns : principles

4.1 For many people, the principal ethical problem raised by xenotransplantation will concern the relationship between human beings and other animals. As described in Chapter 3, xenotransplantation is currently at the research stage. The research involves the use of animals to provide transplant material and also to act as experimental recipients of transplants. Should xenotransplantation develop into a successful clinical procedure it will involve the breeding and killing of animals on a large scale in order to provide organs and tissue for transplantation. In addition, the use of transgenic pigs for xenotransplantation raises questions about the genetic modification of animals to provide organs and tissue.

4.2 The Working Party was charged with examining the ethical issues raised by the use of animals specifically for xenografting. As a first step, the arguments for and against the use of animals for medical purposes **in general** were reviewed. These arguments are summarised briefly in the first part of the chapter. The chapter then goes on to consider whether, even if the use of animals for medical purposes in general is held to be ethically acceptable, there are particular concerns about their use for xenografting. Two issues are discussed:

- the ethical acceptability of the use, respectively, of primates, and of animals other than primates, to supply transplant material;
- the ethical issues raised by the use of genetically modified animals to provide organs for xenotransplantation.

The use of animals for medical purposes

4.3 Many would endorse the view that animals have interests, particularly in the avoidance of suffering, that should be respected, but that in certain limited circumstances those interests may be outweighed by the interests of human beings provided that everything possible is done to minimise distress to the animals. In considering the ethical concerns about the use of animals for xenotransplantation, it was found necessary to explore this view in more detail. For others hold the opinion that all use of animals by human beings for medical purposes is wrong, no matter how great the benefits. The view that there should be an absolute prohibition on the use of animals for medical purposes is a minority position within UK society. It meets an equally conscientiously held view that, in certain circumstances, it is permissible, and perhaps even required, to use animals for human benefit. But justice will not have been done to the importance and complexity of the issues involved if the arguments for and against the use of animals for medical purposes are not reviewed.

4.4 The essence of the problem is that, if animals are to be used for medical purposes in ways that would not be considered ethically acceptable if applied to human beings, then there must be some basis for drawing the distinction between animals and human beings. If there are no convincing reasons to ascribe to animals a lower moral status than that ascribed to human beings, then the use of animals for medical purposes would be hard to justify. In recent years, the argument has been gaining ground that animals should be accorded a higher moral status than has been admitted hitherto. Two distinct philosophical approaches may be used to support this shift in opinion. The first approach starts from the position that the interests of animals, particularly in avoiding suffering, should be taken into account when judging whether it is acceptable to use them for medical purposes that benefit human beings. The second approach argues that animals, like human beings, have rights that must be respected when considering their use for such purposes.

The balance of animal suffering and human benefit

4.5 It is now widely recognised that many animals, and certainly the mammals that would be used for xenografts, are susceptible to pain and suffering. Some argue that there is no logical reason to distinguish morally the pain and suffering felt by animals from that felt by human beings. Suffering is suffering wherever and to whoever it is caused. It would be wrong to weigh animal suffering less heavily than human suffering, just as it would be wrong to weigh the suffering of one human being less heavily than another.[1] This is a utilitarian argument which holds that ethically acceptable actions are those which increase the benefit, or reduce the harm, to as many individuals as possible. When judging the acceptability of the use of animals for xenotransplantation, or for any other medical purpose, a decision must be made about whether the pain and suffering caused to the animals is justified by the potential benefit to the human being.

4.6 In some cases, such as the use of animals for testing cosmetic products used for beauty treatments, there is widespread agreement that the benefit to human beings is trivial and does not warrant the suffering involved. But in other cases, weighing the pain and suffering to animals against the benefit to human beings is not easy. Different people will give different weight to the harms and the benefits and so will come to differing conclusions about the acceptability of using animals for a particular purpose. Despite these difficulties, however, judgements have to be made and the Working

1 Singer P (1995) **Animal Liberation** Second edition. London: Pimlico.

Party accepts the principle that in some cases, the saving of human life or of significantly enhancing its quality may justify a certain amount of animal suffering, provided this is kept to a minimum.

Animal rights

4.7 According to the alternative, rights-based approach, if animals share with human beings some or all of those characteristics that, in the case of human beings, would lead us to assert that they have certain rights, then those rights should be ascribed to the animals as well.[2] The ascription of rights, whether to human beings or animals, rests on the principle that the lives of individuals have an inherent value. Such individuals should be treated as ends in themselves rather than merely as means to the happiness or well-being of others. The British Union for the Abolition of Vivisection wrote in their submission: "*The use of healthy animals as a source of 'spare parts' for humans represents a fundamental denial of the inherent value of those animals' lives.*"

4.8 According to this view, there are fundamental moral constraints on what can be done to those who have rights. Such constraints should not be overridden, no matter how great the benefit accruing to others from so doing. The right to life, for example, dictates that a rights holder, human being or animal, should not be killed, however painlessly, even if countless others could potentially benefit thereby. Similarly, restrictions on the ways in which human beings may be used in medical research should extend to animal rights holders as well. Some argue that any use of animals for medical purposes is a violation of their basic rights, and as such, that it should not be countenanced. Thus, Animal Aid wrote in their submission: "*Animals have value in their own right and do not exist to be harmfully exploited by man.*" The issue of rights, however, remains controversial and is even more so in the case of animal rights. Moreover, it is not necessary to endorse the notion of animal rights in order to conclude that animals should be granted protection against certain procedures.

Self-awareness and personhood

4.9 Whether the argument is framed in terms of the interests or the rights of animals, the crucial point is the extent to which animals share the features supposed to be important to human interests and rights. The feature to which most importance has generally been attached is that of self-awareness.[3] This may be described as the

2 Regan T (1983) **The Case for Animal Rights.** London: Routledge & Kegan Paul.

3 Reviewed in Smith J A and Boyd K M eds. (1991) **Lives in the Balance : The ethics of using animals in biomedical research.** The report of a Working Party of the Institute of Medical Ethics. Oxford: Oxford University Press. In particular pp 319-23.

consciousness an individual has of his or her own condition and experiences. To be self-aware requires a high degree of intelligence, the capacity to make comparisons and judgements, and a language with which to articulate them. Self-awareness allows individuals to plan, to make choices and to engage in complex social relationships. Most significantly, for the purposes of this discussion, it has been argued that suffering and death are uniquely painful to a self-aware being who not only senses pain but can also perceive the damage being done to his or her self and future.

4.10 Individuals that possess these characteristics, founded in self-awareness, may be regarded as persons. Until recently, the moral status of personhood has been supposed to be the unique prerogative of human beings. On these grounds the human being is often regarded as more than a 'mere animal', and the human condition as fundamentally superior to that of animals. In Christian thought, human beings "*have unique significance and value because only they are made in the image of God. (Genesis 1:27)*" [4] In this view, animals would not merit the same moral consideration as human beings, and animal interests would weigh less heavily than human interests. While great weight would be placed on the reduction of animal suffering as an end in itself, the painless killing of animals for the purposes of saving human life or improving its quality would be considered acceptable.

4.11 Recent research into the mental life and intelligence of non-human animals has, however, led to claims that the features qualifying human beings for personhood are also present, to varying degrees, in other species.[5, 6] There is evidence that some animals, notably the higher primates, have much in common with human beings, including self-awareness, complex social relationships and many of the other characteristics that have often been supposed to make human beings unique.[7] If that is so, then these animals should be accorded the same moral status as human beings.

4.12 On the other hand, certain human individuals, whether due to congenital defects, accident or disease, lack the features such as self-awareness and intelligence that are generally taken as criteria for personhood. Thus, the boundaries of personhood and of the human species do not exactly coincide, but rather overlap. Some non-human animals might be considered persons and some human beings might not be considered persons.

---

4 Submission to the Working Party from the Christian Medical Fellowship.

5 Singer P (1995) **Animal Liberation** Second edition. London: Pimlico.

6 Regan T (1983) **The Case for Animal Rights**. London: Routledge & Kegan Paul.

7 Parker S and Gibson K eds. (1990) **"Language" and intelligence in monkeys and apes**. Cambridge: Cambridge University Press.

Speciesism and the moral community

4.13 According to this argument, the capacities of human beings and some non-human animals, such as higher primates, may overlap to such an extent that there is no basis for a distinction of treatment. To deny this implication, it is argued, is simply to draw a distinction on the ground that one individual is of the human species and another is of a non-human species. Such speciesism, some have claimed, is no more acceptable than racism or sexism.[8] Stephen Clark wrote in his submission: "*Till the eighteenth century every civilised society kept human slaves. Those of us who have tried to absorb the implication of Darwinian theory (that species are not natural kinds) suspect that our descendants will be just as critical of our casual contempt for those we know to be our cousins.*" For those who wish to press the charge of speciesism there are two further implications. One is that non-human animals whose capacities match those of human beings should be included within the moral community. A second implication is that it would not be appropriate to include within the moral community human beings whose capacities do not qualify them for personhood. It has been argued, for example, that anencephalic babies, suffering from a fatal neurological condition in which the cerebral hemispheres of the brain are absent, are not persons. Some would regard it as acceptable to use such babies to provide organs for transplantation.[9] It is even argued that to use animals that qualify as persons for medical purposes, rather than human beings that do not, is morally unacceptable.[10]

4.14 This second implication leads many to caution against the use of animals as sources of organs for transplantation, since to do so is to embark upon a 'slippery slope'.[11] Once the use of animals is sanctioned, it is argued, then there can be no principled objections, for example, to the procurement of organs from anencephalic human babies. For many people, the idea that **any** human being could be used in such a way is deeply abhorrent. Similar sentiments underlie the protection, extended to all human beings, from uncontrolled use in medical research, and the prohibition on using organs from human beings except under conditions of consent. It can be argued that vulnerable individuals, such as anencephalic babies, are more deserving of protection not less so.[12] These sentiments are too strong to be easily cast aside.

4.15 Thus the notion of speciesism has to be treated with some caution. Our natural emotional response to, and concern for, members of our own species is clearly built deeply into our nature and it is not clear that the option of responding to members

---

8 Singer P (1995) **Animal Liberation** Second edition. London: Pimlico.

9 British Medical Association's Ethics, Science and Information Division (1993) **Medical Ethics Today: Its practice and philosophy.** London: BMJ Publishing Group. p 27.

10 Frey R G (1987) Animal Parts, Human Wholes : On the use of animals as a source of organs for human transplants. **Biomedical Ethics Reviews,** pp 89-107.

11 A point made by Meg Stacey in her submission to the Working Party.

12 A point made by Jeremy Caddick in his submission to the Working Party.

of other species, with the same concern in every case, is open to us. We should consider therefore what our treatment of non-human animals should be in its own terms, rather than in terms of consistency with our treatment of human beings.

Relationships

4.16 Arguably the moral status of human beings depends not only on their individual capacities but also on the histories of their relationships with others. Thus, although an anencephalic baby might be considered to lack the capacities or potentials necessary for personhood, it is nevertheless bound to particular human parents and, through them, to a wider set of people, in deep networks of emotion and attachment. These relationships with parents and others would draw it into the moral community. In general, then, human beings cannot be understood or treated as though each were an isolated, self-contained entity, whose rights and responsibilities, or well-being and suffering, could be assessed independently of his or her involvement with others.

4.17 This argument could apply, moreover, not only to relationships among human beings but also to relationships between human beings and animals. In this context it is important to distinguish between **relationship** and **relatedness**. It might be expected that the non-human animals most likely to have the capacities necessary for personhood, and therefore to be eligible for inclusion within the moral community, would be individuals of species most closely related to humankind - above all, higher primates such as chimpanzees and baboons. In practice, however, we may be more ready to include familiar, domestic animals than unfamiliar primates, even though the latter are much closer to human beings in a biological sense. This is because the personhood of the animal is seen to derive from its involvement with human beings (most obvious in the case of pets), rather than from its underlying genetic relatedness to human beings. When relationships are taken into account, pet dogs or cats, or indeed farm animals such as pigs, may well seem more person-like than baboons or chimpanzees. This is reflected in the special legal protection extended to dogs, cats and horses, as well as primates, in the UK.[13]

4.18 Animals may also form relationships among themselves. Just as in assessing the well-being or suffering of human beings it is necessary to take into account their relationships with others, the same may be true in the case of animals as well. A chimpanzee mother suffers grief at the loss of her offspring: to harm her offspring causes harm to the mother. If animals are to be killed to provide organs for transplantation, or otherwise used for medical purposes, and if these animals form social relationships with one another, then the pain and suffering caused to others by the harm done to an individual animal cannot be disregarded.

13 Animal (Scientific Procedures) Act 1986 : Section 10.

Attitudes to nature

4.19 Arguments for and against the use of animals for medical purposes also have to be placed in the context of differing views about the relationship of human beings to nature in general. Those who favour using animals in medicine have been accused by their opponents of adopting a wholly instrumental attitude towards nature, and of failing to recognise that human beings are part of the natural world and have responsibilities for it. The Genetics Forum wrote in their submission: "*The use of animals as sources of cells, tissues and organs for humans causes us much concern. It encourages the concept of animals as 'pharm' factories and reinforces the ethos that they merely exist in order to satisfy human needs.*"

4.20 As an alternative, critics advocate a concept of stewardship, according to which human beings should not seek to dominate nature but should instead stand in a relationship of care and concern for its continued flourishing. Another, not incompatible, view is that human beings should see themselves not as separate from nature but as a small part of a larger world.[14] For some people, these views would be compatible with the limited use of animals in medical procedures where the benefit was clear, demonstrable and large. For others, these views might entail a direct prohibition on the use of animals for medical purposes. The argument might turn, in part, upon scale. Thus, it might be held that the limited use of animals in current medical procedures does not abuse the human relationship with nature. But procedures involving the use of animals on a large scale, such as xenotransplantation if it were successful, would be unacceptable.

4.21 Another element of this argument might depend on a distinction between customary and new practices. New uses of animals might be objectionable in the way that existing uses, provided that they are not cruel, are not. In their submission to the Working Party, the Farmers' Forum (a discussion group of Christian farmers) expressed an objection to rearing animals solely for the purposes of xenotransplantation. For some, a completely new use of animals, such as for xenografting, might be unacceptable, whereas if that use developed from, and was continuous with, an established use of animals, then it might be more acceptable. It is important not simply to be prejudiced against innovation, however, and some would question the ethical acceptability of established practices involving animals, such as eating meat. The Church of Scotland pointed out in their submission: "*There is also a 'naturalness' argument here. It is a basic fact of life that everyone has to eat to live. We may debate whether eating animals by humans is acceptable, but it is clearly 'natural' in the sense that many animals are also carnivores. It is not 'natural' to use an animal as spare parts. It is human artifice. That is not to say it is wrong, but it is not the same as eating an animal.*" [15]

---

14 Goodin R E (1992) **Green Political Theory**. Cambridge: Polity Press.

15 Submission to the Working Party from the Working Group on Genetic Engineering in Non-human Life Forms of the Society, Religion & Technology Project of the Church of Scotland.

4.22 How far should public policy be based on concerns about the underlying attitudes that the development of a particular technology is thought to reveal? If human beings have not got their relationship with the rest of nature right, and if there is continual unjustifiable exploitation of other species for human use, then it would be wrong to allow the development of a new technology that increased this exploitation. Innovation may be undertaken for a variety of motives, however, and it is not easy to determine, from people's actions, what their attitudes are. But there is undoubted force in the moral argument that rests upon the question: what sort of people do our social and technical practices reveal us to be? If we do not like what we see when we look honestly in the mirror, then there is cause for thought at least.

Conscientious objections to the use of animals for medical purposes

4.23 Some people may oppose the use of animals for medical purposes because of particular religious or metaphysical views. For example, the Jain Academy wrote that *"Jains are against all animal experimentation and use of animal cells, tissues and organs, as it is against all the principles of reverence for life and non-violence."* Where convictions of this kind rest upon metaphysical assumptions that are not widely shared, they cannot easily be made the basis of public policy. People's opinions about the use of animals for medical purposes, whether or not articulated in the name of a religious faith, are highly diverse, as the submissions received by the Working Party reveal. The Medical Ethics Group of the Reform Synagogues of Great Britain wrote in their submission: *"Yet whereas we are expected to do everything possible to prevent [animal] suffering there is no doubt that our duty to human beings outweighs that to animals".*

4.24 A more specific issue is raised by the proposed use of pigs for xenotransplantation. Would the use of animals regarded as ritually unclean be ethically acceptable? The Chairman of the Sharia Council has explained that under Islamic law, while eating pigs is forbidden, other uses can be assumed to be permitted.[16] Indeed, even eating pigs is permitted if this is necessary to save life. Similarly, the Reform Synagogues of Great Britain indicated in their submission to the Working Party that the mainstream Jewish authorities would accept the use of pigs in order to save life. Thus, xenotransplantation of pig organs and tissue, as a life-preserving treatment, would be acceptable. Nevertheless, some people viewing pigs as unclean may have objections to their use for xenotransplantation. The Union of Muslim Organisations of UK and Eire wrote in their submission that xenografts *"might be allowed provided the animal used is not a pig or other prohibited animal"*. Thus, there may be, quite legitimately, a range of positions with regard to xenotransplantation even within one

16 Zaki Badawi explains the Islamic position. **The Guardian**, 25 August 1995.

religion. These diverse opinions highlight the importance of taking account of different attitudes towards xenotransplantation. This issue is discussed further in Chapter 7 (paragraph 7.27 - 7.33).

The use of animals for medical purposes: conclusions

4.25 The ethical issues raised by the use of animals in medical research are complicated and, in this chapter, the arguments are briefly reviewed. The issues have been discussed at length in the book **Lives in the Balance: The ethics of using animals in biomedical research** [17] produced by a Working Party of the Institute of Medical Ethics. That Working Party produced the following statement:

> "*The Working Party contains a variety of views on the moral status of animals but is prepared to accept for the present that biomedical research using animal subjects is justified as an undesirable but unavoidable necessity. This working agreement extends to the following points:*
>
> *1 In the absence of any scientifically and morally acceptable alternative, some use of animals in biomedical research can be justified as necessary to safeguard and improve the health and alleviate the suffering of human beings and animals.*
>
> *2 The benefits, in turn, depend on the advancement of fundamental scientific knowledge but even when no therapeutic or other practical benefit can yet be derived from it, any significant advance in scientific knowledge is a good, and **may** serve as a justification for using animals to that end.*
>
> *3 However, not every projected improvement to human health or addition to scientific knowledge is sufficiently significant to justify every use of animals. Some uses of animals may have adverse effects too serious to justify them at all, while in other cases the adverse effects may be considered disproportionately serious in relation to the significance of the results gained.*
>
> *4 In the latter case especially, both the potential benefits of a particular research project and the likelihood of the project achieving those benefits need to be assessed carefully before they, in turn, are weighed against the likely adverse effects to the animals.*"

17 Smith J A and Boyd K M eds. (1991) **Lives in the Balance : The ethics of using animals in biomedical research.** The Report of a Working Party of the Institute of Medical Ethics. Oxford: Oxford University Press. pp 310-11.

4.26 All members of the present Working Party are prepared to accept the statement of the Institute of Medical Ethics Working Party, though they differ in the detailed interpretation of the judgements implied in them. Another Committee, which examined the ethical implications of emerging technologies in the breeding of farm animals, reached similar conclusions, stating that the use of animals is permissible providing that use is humane, but that "*harms of a certain degree and kind ought under no circumstances to be inflicted on an animal.*"[18] Of paramount importance is the need to keep to a minimum any suffering or pain experienced by the animals. This is discussed at length in Chapter 5. It is also important to keep the number of animals used to a minimum, and to find alternatives to the use of animals where possible.

4.27 For those who do not accept the use of animals for medical purposes, xenotransplantation will, in principle, be unacceptable. The Working Party does not take this view and considers that some use of animals for xenotransplantation can be justified in principle. There are specific issues, however, that need further consideration. In what follows the particular ethical implications of the use of primates for xenotransplantation are considered. Attention has focused on the pig as an alternative to the use of primates for xenotransplantation (paragraph 3.4). In the final part of this chapter the ethical issues associated with the use of pigs for xenotransplantation are discussed, including those issues arising from their genetic modification for this purpose (paragraphs 4.42 - 4.54).

Concerns about the use of primates for xenotransplantation

4.28 Because of the genetic closeness of higher primates to human beings, their organs and tissue are likely to offer a good chance of success for xenotransplantation (paragraphs 3.18 - 3.20). With a suitable immunosuppressant drug regime, it may become possible to transplant primate organs and tissues reliably and effectively. If xenotransplantation using primate organs and tissue subsequently became widespread, this would represent a significant and new way of using primates. Currently, in the UK, the use of primates is very strictly controlled with only very small numbers being used for research purposes (paragraphs 4.37). Thus, to breed primates on a large scale would be contrary to currently accepted practice in the UK. As such, the ethical issues raised by the use of primates for xenotransplantation require exploring in some detail.

4.29 The very reason that makes primates appear to be well suited for transplantation, namely their evolutionary relatedness to human beings, also leads many people to think that it would be wrong to use them for this purpose. A simplified diagram showing the evolutionary relationships between different primate species is shown in Figure 4.1.

---

18 Banner M (Chairman) (1995) **Report of the Committee to Consider the Ethical Implications of Emerging Technologies in the Breeding of Farm Animals.** London: HMSO. p 1.

Figure 4.1 The evolutionary relationships between primate species[19]

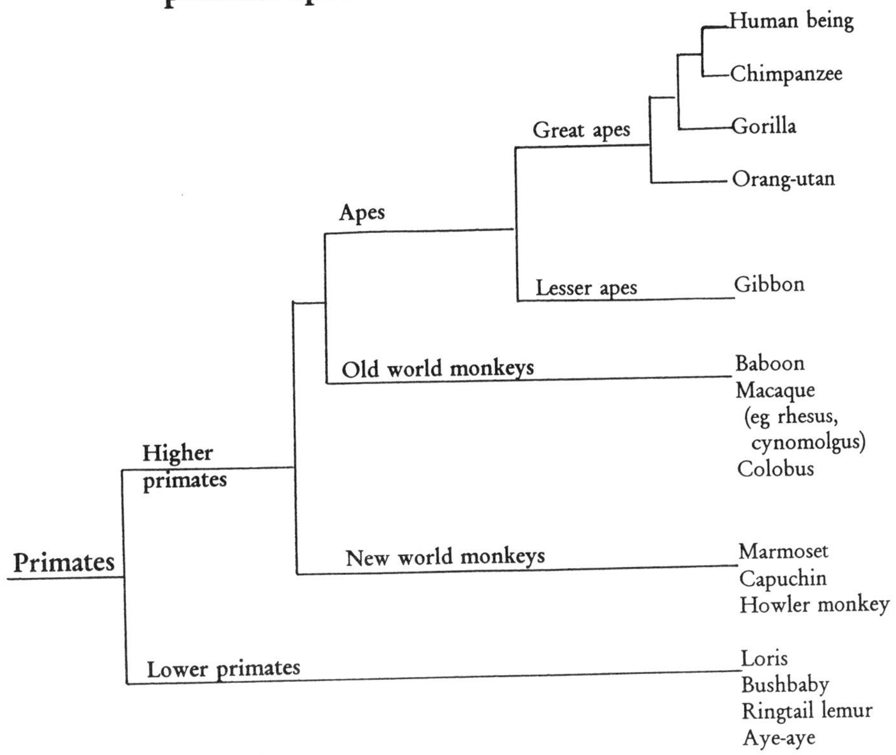

The characteristics, for example, of intelligence and complex social interactions, of these closely related higher primates appear to be so like those of human beings that using members of those species as sources for xenotransplantation might well be seen as ethically unacceptable. Many have argued that the same concern should be extended to higher primates as is extended to human beings. The question then is how far this concern should extend. The close evolutionary relationship of higher primates with human beings suggests that they will share the capacity for self-awareness to the highest degree, and there is good scientific evidence that this is the case. Some would argue, however, that any ethical reservations about using higher primates for xenotransplantation should apply much more broadly. Many non-primate species, possibly including pigs, display comparable capacities of intelligence and sociality, albeit in forms that less closely resemble the human and thus appeal less strongly to human moral sensibility. To limit reservations to those species closest to human beings, in this view, is to be swayed by sentimental anthropomorphism.

19 Adapted from Byrne R (1995) **The Thinking Ape : evolutionary origins of intelligence.** Oxford: Oxford University Press.

4.30 Contrary to both the above positions, there is a view that, notwithstanding the features that primates (or other species) share with human beings, it would still be wrong not to save a human life even if the price of so doing was the life of a primate. According to this position, human life has the greater value, and therefore the primate's life can be legitimately sacrificed.

4.31 It is difficult to know what sort of argument would resolve this disagreement of value. For the question is whether there is sufficient likeness between human beings and other primates for the same constraints to be imposed upon the use of primates as are imposed upon human beings. This question of likeness is not amenable to empirical resolution, but is one of fundamental moral judgement. The difficulty of resolving the issue is reflected in the diversity of opinions that people hold on the matter. Some consider that there is sufficient difference between the moral value of human life and the value of higher primate life to make the use of the latter acceptable in certain circumstances. Yet many who take this view would nevertheless argue that higher primates should be used only in very restricted and carefully controlled circumstances and only if, for example, the use of pigs for xenotransplantation turned out not to be possible. Others argue that the resemblance between human beings and species like chimpanzees and baboons is too close to justify the use of such primates as a source of material for xenotransplantation. Yet many of these people would accept that no clear boundary separates animals whose use is acceptable from those whose use is not acceptable. This dilemma concerning the moral distinction between human beings and primates is extremely difficult to resolve. In addition to this fundamental judgement of value, however, there are a number of other considerations that contribute to determining the ethical acceptability of using primates to provide organs for xenotransplantation. These are discussed below.

Welfare

4.32 The similarities in behaviour between human beings and other primates may not lead to a consensus about their relative moral status. But they undoubtedly highlight the importance of welfare considerations in the use of primates for xenotransplantation. The routine breeding and maintenance of animals free from infectious organisms might require birth by Caesarean section, rearing in isolation, and repeated monitoring to assess levels of infection (paragraphs 5.18 - 5.22). The intelligent and social nature of primates would make such conditions particularly severe for them.

Conservation

4.33 In the case of chimpanzees, which are an endangered species, strong conservationist concerns suggest that their use for xenotransplantation should be forbidden. While chimpanzees have been used to provide organs for xenotransplantation in the past, there is now an international consensus within the xenotransplantation community that the use of chimpanzees for providing organs is unacceptable on conservation grounds alone.

4.34 Conservation concerns do not currently apply to baboons, which are not endangered at present, and which are, in fact, regarded as a pest in many parts of the world. Might baboons become endangered if they were to be used as a source of organs for xenotransplantation? Capture of wild baboons for use as a source of organs is unlikely because of the need to ensure that the animals used for xenotransplantation are free of disease (Chapter 6). Like all primates, however, baboons breed slowly, with breeding females producing a maximum of one offspring every 15 months.[20] Because of this slow rate of reproduction, the current colonies of baboons would probably not be able to provide sufficient numbers with which to establish breeding colonies of disease-free baboons to supply organs for xenotransplantation. It would be necessary to capture wild baboons to augment these breeding colonies.

4.35 In contrast to chimpanzees, baboons are relatively easy to catch and transport. They also adapt well to captivity and breeding colonies are not difficult to establish. With the unmet demand for organs for transplantation in the US alone estimated to be 100,000 every year,[21] however, establishing breeding colonies of baboons to provide organs for transplantation would require the capture of large numbers of animals. Hence, although baboons are abundant at present, their use to provide organs for xenotransplantation might have a significant effect on their numbers. It should also be borne in mind that deforestation is destroying the natural habitat of all primates. Baboons, being tough and adaptable, can survive in other habitats, but large-scale capture for xenotransplantation would be one more pressure. Moreover, it is possible that, if xenotransplantation involving baboons were seen to be successful, there would be renewed interest in attempts to use chimpanzees for xenotransplantation. This might lead to increased pressure on the endangered chimpanzee population.

---

20 Whitney R A and Wickings E J (1987) Macaques and other old world simians, Chapter 40 of **The UFAW Handbook on the Care and Management of Laboratory Animals** Sixth Edition. UK: Longman Scientific & Technical.

21 From the belly of the beast. **The Economist**, 21 October 1995, pp 137-9.

Safety

4.36 The safety of the use of primate organs and tissue for xenotransplantation must also be considered. A risk associated with the transplantation of animal organs or tissue into human beings is that infectious organisms will also be transmitted into the human population, leading to the emergence of new diseases. Because of the biological similarity between human beings and other primates, the risk that infectious organisms from a primate will be able to infect and cause disease in human beings is greater than the risk of disease transmission from, say, pigs to human beings. There is evidence that infectious organisms do, indeed, pass from primates to human beings and cause disease.[22] This suggests that a cautious attitude should be adopted to xenotransplantation involving primates (paragraphs 6.10 - 6.12).

The use of primates for xenotransplantation: conclusions

4.37 Serious ethical concerns are raised by the possible use of primates for xenotransplantation. The sophisticated capacities of primates suggest that any harm suffered by them should be given great weight. This position is reflected in the principles underlying current practice in the UK. Wherever possible, primates used for medical purposes must be purpose-bred.[23] Very few licences allowing primate use are awarded: only 29 in 1994. The use of wild-caught primates for medical purposes requires "*exceptional and specific justification*".[24] **The Working Party endorses the special protection afforded to higher primates used for medical and scientific purposes.**

4.38 The Working Party would accept the use of very small numbers of primates **as recipients of organs** for research during the development of xenotransplantation using non-primate animals as sources of organs. In this case, the harm caused by using a small number of primates for research into xenotransplantation, while undesirable, can be justified by the potential benefits if xenotransplantation were to become a successful procedure.

4.39 The routine use of higher primates to supply organs for xenotransplantation on a scale sufficient to meet the organ shortage would represent a new use of primates in the UK. In contrast to the use of primates for research purposes, this would entail the use of relatively large numbers of animals, not for a short period during the development of a procedure, but for the long term. As discussed above, in addition to the special weight given to the harm suffered by primates, additional concerns

---

22 Allan J S (1995) Xenotransplantation at a crossroads: Prevention versus progress. **Nature Medicine**, 2: 18-21.

23 Animals (Scientific Procedures) Act 1986: Section 7.

24 **Report of the Animal Procedures Committee for 1994** (1995) London: HMSO Cm 2996, p 7.

must be taken into account. The potential risk of extinction, even to species like the baboon that are not currently endangered, must be taken seriously. Xenotransplantation using primate organs or tissue may pose particular risks of disease transmission.

4.40 Given the ethical concerns raised by the use of primates for xenotransplantation, attention has turned to developing the pig as an alternative source of organs and tissue. As discussed below, in the view of the Working Party, the use of pigs for xenotransplantation raises fewer ethical concerns. To develop the use of primates for xenotransplantation, when there is an ethically acceptable alternative, would not be justifiable. **The Working Party recommends that non-primate species should be regarded as the source animals of choice for xenotransplantation.** However, possibilities for alleviating the organ shortage which do not involve the use of animals, such as increased donation of human organs and the development of artificial organs and tissue, should be actively pursued.

4.41 The Working Party would like to draw attention to a longer-term issue. It is possible that, after a number of years of research, it would be found that the use of pigs could not deliver effective, reliable and safe organs and tissue for transplantation. Would it then be ethically acceptable to use primate organs and tissue for xenotransplantation? The members of the Working Party were agreed that the use of primates would be ethically **unacceptable** if **any** of the following conditions obtained:

- improving the supply of human organs and tissue and the use of alternatives, such as mechanical organs and tissue replacement, could meet the organ shortage;
- the use of higher primates would result in them becoming an endangered species;
- concerns about the possible transmission of disease from higher primates to human beings could not be met; or
- the welfare of the animals could not be maintained to a high standard.

These conditions would rule out all use of chimpanzees on conservation grounds. When considering the hypothetical situation in which the conditions might be satisfied for a species such as the baboon, the members of the Working Party found that their opinions did not coincide on what would be the correct course. Some felt that the use of primates to supply organs for xenotransplantation would never be acceptable. Other members of the Working Party felt that, should these circumstances come to prevail, it would be appropriate to reconsider the use of higher primates to supply organs for xenotransplantation. This division of opinion may reflect an ethical dilemma that is currently unresolved for many people.

The use of pigs for xenotransplantation

4.42 The main alternative to using primates for xenotransplantation is to use pigs (paragraph 3.4). Thus, the moral justification for using pigs to provide organs for xenotransplantation must be considered. When considering the use of primates for xenotransplantation, the capacities they share with human beings, notably their self-awareness, led to ethical concerns about their use for xenotransplantation. While unquestionably intelligent and sociable animals,[25] there is less evidence that pigs share capacities with human beings to the extent that primates do. As such, the adverse effects suffered by the pigs used to supply organs for xenotransplantation would not outweigh the potential benefits to human beings. In the UK, the breeding of pigs for human use is well established. It is difficult to see how, in a society in which the breeding of pigs for food and clothing is accepted, their use for life-saving medical procedures such as xenotransplantation could be unacceptable. **The Working Party concluded that the use of pigs for the routine supply of organs for xenotransplantation was ethically acceptable.**

4.43 In order for it to be ethically acceptable to use pigs for xenotransplantation it will be necessary to ensure that the conditions in which they are bred and reared are of the highest possible standard from the point of view of welfare, and that any pain and suffering is kept to a minimum. Animal welfare issues are discussed in Chapter 5.

4.44 If pigs are to be used for xenotransplantation, they are likely to have been modified so that they contain genetic material of human origin (paragraphs 3.24 - 3.32). The next section discusses the ethical concerns that may arise from the use of transgenic animals for xenografting.

The use of transgenic animals for xenotransplantation

4.45 The essence of transgenesis is that a gene from one species is incorporated into another. The transferred gene enables the transgenic animal to produce a particular protein. The transgenic pigs bred for xenotransplantation contain a human gene which produces a complement regulating protein. This reduces the immune response to transplanted organs (paragraphs 3.24 - 3.29). It is around the transfer of genetic material that ethical concerns turn. One UK study, of schoolchildren aged 14 - 16, found that they were particularly concerned about genetic modification of farm animals.[26] Some see the production of transgenic animals as an unnatural act that attempts to change the nature of animals and violates species boundaries. According to this view, genes have a particular significance because they contain the information

25 Singer P (1995) **Animal Liberation** Second edition. London: Pimlico. pp 119-29.

26 Lock R and Miles C (1993) Biotechnology and genetic engineering: students' knowledge and attitudes. **Journal of Biological Education**, 27, 267-72.

that determines the essence of any one species. To move genes around is to destroy the integrity of species as natural kinds, and to create unnatural hybrids. Within the Judaeo-Christian tradition human beings are seen as being created in the image of God which leads, for some, to a specific objection to experimentation using God-like human genes.[27] For others such "*'mutilation' of the human body*" would be sanctioned in the interests of saving life.[28] A number of arguments, however, suggest that the production of transgenic animals need not be viewed as a drastic or unnatural procedure. The issues have been thoroughly examined by two committees set up by the Ministry of Agriculture, Fish and Food.[29, 30]

4.46 First, species boundaries are not, in fact, inviolate, but change as evolution occurs. Some regard transgenic techniques as no more than an extension of traditional breeding techniques that artificially produce new animal breeds.[31] There is also evidence that, at a low level, the transfer of genetic material from one species to another occurs naturally. For example, genetic material may be transferred between different types of bacteria. Some would question whether there is any significant qualitative difference between this type of event and the transfer of genetic material from human beings into pigs.

4.47 Second, it can be questioned whether genes of human origin represent particular elements of essential humanity. It is only in combination with all the other genes that make up the human genome that a particular gene contributes to the specification of features characteristic of the human species. Considered in isolation, therefore, there is nothing specifically human about a gene that has been obtained from a human source. Similarly, genes obtained from an animal species do not have to be seen as representing a particular element of that animal. If this view is adopted, the transfer of a gene from one species to another is far less significant. In addition, because of the technology involved, the genetic material actually transferred to a transgenic animal is almost certain to be a copy of the gene rather than the original gene that was obtained from the organism.[32]

4.48 In addition, many transgenic animals are modified on a very small scale and in a very specific way. Consider the production of transgenic pigs to supply organs for xenotransplantation. At present, it is unlikely that more than one or two genes of

27 A view set out by R Gill in his submission to the Working Party.

28 Submission of the Reform Synagogues of Great Britain.

29 Polkinghorne J (Chairman) (1993) **Report of the Committee on the Ethics of Genetic Modification and Food Use.** London: HMSO.

30 Banner M (Chairman) (1995) **Report of the Committee to Consider the Ethical Implications of Emerging Technologies in the Breeding of Farm Animals.** London: HMSO.

31 A point made in the submission from the Church in Wales.

32 Polkinghorne J (Chairman) (1993) **Report of the Committee on the Ethics of Genetic Modification and Food Use.** London: HMSO, pp 5-6.

human origin will be incorporated into transgenic pigs. Since the pig genome probably contains in the order of 50,000 - 100,000 genes, this is proportionately a very small change.[33] In addition, the human genes contain information that will make only a very minor and specific alteration to the surface antigens of the pig's cells (paragraph 3.25). The physical appearance and characteristics of the pig will not change in any measurable sense. Will the nature of the pig change in any way that is ethically important? For the reasons set out above, the Working Party does not consider that the introduction of very small numbers of human genes into transgenic pigs makes the pigs in any sense human or creates a hybrid species. Similar conclusions were reached by both the Polkinghorne and the Banner Committees. Inserting small quantities of genetic material of human origin was not thought to make an animal in any sense human. The Banner Committee concluded that procedures that failed "*to respect the natural characteristics, dignity and worth of animals*" would be objectionable.[34] While this might rule out the use of transgenesis to produce pigs with altered behaviour, for example reduced sentience, the Banner Committee considered the production of transgenic pigs for xenotransplantation acceptable. The Polkinghorne Committee reported that, for many people, whether genetic modification is acceptable would depend on whether it was intended to preserve or enhance human life.[35] By this criterion the production of transgenic pigs to provide organs for xenotransplantation would be acceptable.

4.49 In the light of the arguments discussed above, **the Working Party concluded that the use of transgenic pigs that have been genetically modified to reduce the human immune response to pig organs was ethically acceptable.** As with any use of animals for medical purposes, it is important that the welfare of transgenic animals is not unacceptably compromised. This is of particular concern in the context of transgenesis because some of the transgenic animals produced to date have suffered from ill effects. One example is the introduction of growth genes into pigs in order to make them grow faster for food production. The animals suffered from a variety of conditions such as arthritis, ulcers and diabetes.[36] There is no evidence to date that the welfare of transgenic pigs developed for xenotransplantation is adversely affected.[37] It is important, however, to be vigilant in assessing the effects of transgenesis on animal welfare. Monitoring the welfare of transgenic pigs for xenotransplantation is discussed in Chapter 5 (paragraphs 5.9 - 5.17).

---

33 Polkinghorne J (Chairman) (1993) **Report of the Committee on the Ethics of Genetic Modification and Food Use.** London: HMSO, p 9.

34 Banner M (Chairman) (1995) **Report of the Committee to Consider the Ethical Implications of Emerging Technologies in the Breeding of Farm Animals.** London: HMSO, p 1.

35 Polkinghorne J (Chairman) (1993) **Report of the Committee on the Ethics of Genetic Modification and Food Use.** London: HMSO, p 9.

36 Reiss M and Straughan R (1996) **Improving Nature? The science and ethics of genetic engineering.** Cambridge: Cambridge University Press.

37 Cozzi E and White D J G (1995) The generation of transgenic pigs as potential organ donors for humans. **Nature Medicine,** 1:964-6.

4.50 Considerable concern about transgenic organisms has turned on the potential risks to the environment should they escape or be released. Some organisms, such as micro-organisms, are not easily contained. Other organisms may have advantages over their unmodified counterparts: for example, transgenic salmon have been produced that grow much faster than unmodified salmon. Initially, at least, transgenic pigs produced for xenotransplantation are likely to be few in number, commercially valuable, relatively easily contained, and with no growth advantage over unmodified pigs. This means that they are unlikely to be made commercially available on the general agricultural market, to escape, or to cause problems if they do escape. Should xenotransplantation become more widespread, it is possible that surpluses of transgenic pigs may arise, and at this point, whether or not they should be made available on the general agricultural market may become an issue.

4.51 The production of transgenic animals is regulated by the Animals (Scientific Procedures) Act 1986 (paragraphs 5.2 - 5.4). To date, relatively few strains of transgenic farm animals have been produced, and none of them have been released from the control of the Act. Were any transgenic animals to be released from control of the Act, a regulatory framework is in place to control the release of genetically modified organisms into the environment. The Advisory Committee on Genetic Modification and the Advisory Committee on Releases to the Environment would advise on such matters. The Genetically Modified Organisms (Deliberate Release) Regulations 1992 and 1993 would require that consent is obtained from the Department of the Environment before transgenic animals were made available or sold, and the Health and Safety Executive would require notification.[38]

4.52 The most likely purpose of making surplus transgenic pigs available on the general agricultural market would be their sale for food. The Polkinghorne Committee concluded that it was acceptable that surplus transgenic animals produced for medical purposes should be used as food rather than discarded needlessly.[39] Both the Advisory Committee on Novel Foods and Processes, and the Food Advisory Committee would advise on the use for food of transgenic pigs produced for xenotransplantation. Should the food use of transgenic pigs or other farm animals be approved, labelling would be required to allow consumers to exercise choice about whether they eat food from genetically modified animals.

4.53 Should their organs and tissue be effective for xenotransplantation, applications may be made to patent transgenic pig strains. There has been much discussion about whether patenting transgenic animals is ethical, and whether it is legal under current patent law.[40] In Europe, patent law is governed by the European Patent

38 Health & Safety (Genetic Manipulation) Regulations (1978).

39 Polkinghorne J (Chairman) (1993) **Report of the Committee on the Ethics of Genetic Modification and Food Use.** London: HMSO, p 15.

40 Is this the work of man or nature? **Independent**, 20 November 1995.

Convention and patents are granted by the European Patent Office. In 1992, the European Patent Office granted a patent for the Harvard Oncomouse, a transgenic mouse strain that has been genetically modified so that it has a predisposition to cancer. The decision provoked widespread protests from animal welfare and environmentalist groups and the European Patent Office has heard evidence relating to 17 different appeals against the patent.[41] The verdict on the appeals is still awaited. At the same time, the European Commission is trying to clarify the situation with a directive that would allow patents on genetically altered animals and plants.[42] The directive has been submitted to the Council of Ministers and the European Parliament for their approval, but a similar directive has previously been rejected by the Parliament.

4.54 A detailed discussion of the ethics of patenting transgenic animals lies outside the scope of this report. The issues have been examined in some detail in a previous report of the Nuffield Council on Bioethics, and elsewhere.[43,44] Proposals to patent transgenic pigs produced for xenotransplantation would increase the debate about the morality and legality of patenting transgenic animals. This adds force to the recommendation of the Nuffield Council in their previous report "*that the Government joins with other member states of the European Patent Convention (EPC) in adopting a protocol to the EPC which would set out in some detail the criteria to be used by national courts when applying the immorality exclusion to patents in the area of human and animal tissue.*" [43]

41 Oncomouse hearing ends up in confusion (1995) **Nature,** 378:427.

42 European proposal reopens debate over patenting of human genes (1995) **Nature,** 378:765.

43 Nuffield Council on Bioethics (1995) Patent Issues, Chapter 11 in **Human Tissue : Ethical and Legal Issues.**

44 National Academies Policy Advisory Group (1995) **Intellectual Property & the Academic Community.**

Chapter 5

Animal concerns : practice

5.1 In Chapter 4 the principles underlying the use of animals for medical purposes in general, and for xenografting in particular, were discussed. The Working Party concluded that the use of transgenic pigs as a source of organs for xenotransplantation was ethically acceptable, provided animal welfare was a high priority. Much stronger ethical concerns are raised by the proposed use of primates to supply organs. The Working Party concluded that non-primate species should be regarded as the source animals of choice for xenotransplantation, but it considered the use of small numbers of primates for research purposes during the development of xenografts was ethically acceptable. In all cases, great attention should be paid to the welfare of any animals used. This chapter looks at the practical implications of these conclusions. The relevant areas of concern are:

- the care of primates used in xenotransplantation research;
- the production and care of transgenic pigs;
- the production of transgenic pigs free from infectious organisms; and
- the removal from transgenic pigs of tissues and organs for xenotransplantation.

In the UK, the use of animals for experimental or other scientific purposes is regulated by the Animals (Scientific Procedures) Act 1986. This chapter describes the protection given to animals by the 1986 Act, and assesses how far it would cover the use of animals for xenotransplantation. The need for any changes is discussed.

Animals (Scientific Procedures) Act 1986

5.2 The Animals (Scientific Procedures) Act 1986 (hereafter called the 1986 Act) and its associated Guidance and Codes of Practice controls the use of animals for scientific purposes in the UK.[1] An animal is defined as any living vertebrate (including fetuses more than 50 per cent of the way through gestation) and one invertebrate -

1 **Home Office Guidance on the Operation of the Animals (Scientific Procedures) Act 1986.** London: HMSO 182 (1990). **Home Office Code of Practice for the Housing and Care of Animals in Designated Breeding and Supplying Establishments.** London: HMSO (1995). **Home Office Code of Practice for the Housing and Care of Animals Used in Scientific Procedures.** London: HMSO 107 (1989).

the common octopus.[2] A scientific procedure is defined as a procedure *"which may have the effect of causing that animal pain, suffering, distress or lasting harm."* [3] Procedures that cause no harm, are outside the Act. Furthermore, the purpose of the work has to be one specified by the 1986 Act. One of these purposes is *"the prevention (whether by the testing of any product or otherwise) or the diagnosis or treatment, of disease, ill-health or abnormality, or their effects, in man, animals or plants."* [4] If a person carries out work that contravenes the requirements of the 1986 Act, he or she may be prosecuted.

5.3 Three forms of control are in operation:

- establishments where scientific procedures are performed on animals must be designated;
- individuals must hold personal licences authorising them to perform certain scientific procedures on animals; and
- project licences must be granted for each specific project using animals.

Before granting a project licence under the 1986 Act, the Secretary of State has to weigh the likely adverse effects on the animals against the benefits likely to accrue as a result of the programme specified in the licence.[5] The Home Secretary is advised by the Home Office Inspectorate which makes decisions on a case-by-case basis. In weighing adverse effects consideration is given to pain, suffering, distress and lasting harm. Three additional criteria are employed: it must be shown that the same aim could not be achieved without the use of animals;[6] the numbers of animals must be kept to a minimum; and the pain and suffering involved must be minimised.[7] The Home Office Inspectorate is also responsible for monitoring approved projects and the individuals and establishments performing regulated procedures.

5.4 The Animal Procedures Committee, a statutory body set up under the 1986 Act, advises the Home Secretary on matters of policy and practice relating to the use of animals for scientific procedures. In certain areas, such as the use of animals for microsurgery, for tobacco research and for cosmetics testing, the Animal Procedures Committee advises on all applications for project licences.[8]

---

2 Animal (Scientific Procedures) Act 1986 : Section 1, amended in 1990 to include *Octopus vulgaris.*

3 Animal (Scientific Procedures) Act 1986 : Section 2.(1).

4 Animals (Scientific Procedures) Act 1986 : Section 5.(3)(a).

5 Animals (Scientific Procedures) Act 1986 : Section 5.(4).

6 Animals (Scientific Procedures) Act 1986 : Section 5.(5).

7 Animals (Scientific Procedures) Act 1986 : Section 10.(2)(a).

8 **Report of the Animal Procedures Committee for 1987** (1988) London: HMSO, pp 8 - 10.

5.5 Any decision, therefore, about the use of animals for medical purposes will be made by the Home Office Inspectorate, in consultation, where necessary, with the Animal Procedures Committee. In principle, the use of animals for xenotransplantation would come within the control of the 1986 Act, since the aim would be the "*treatment of disease, ill health or abnormality in man and animals.*" As set out below, the use of animals for xenotransplantation raises questions about their breeding, especially if they are genetically modified, the welfare implications of producing animals free from infectious organisms, and their slaughter. The discussion in Chapter 4 indicated how difficult it is to reach decisions about the ethical use of animals. **The Working Party recommends that the convention by which the Animal Procedures Committee advises on project licences in difficult areas should extend to applications for the use of animals for xenotransplantation.** When weighing the possible adverse effects on the animals against the likely benefits, the ethical issues discussed in Chapter 4 should be taken into account. It is not clear, however, whether when the 1986 Act is applied in practice all aspects of the use of animals for xenotransplantation will come under, and remain within, its control. For animals not protected by the 1986 Act the same high welfare standards will not apply. This issue and its implications are discussed below.

The care of primates

5.6 Small numbers of primates have already been used to evaluate xenografting from transgenic pigs into a higher primate and this research is likely to continue. Primates are afforded special protection by the 1986 Act.[9] Schedule 2 of the 1986 Act states that primates must be purpose bred for research wherever possible and Home Office policy has been significantly strengthened in this area. A Primate Working Group of the Animal Procedures Committee receives information on all new project licences allowing the use of primates and is consulted about licence applications involving procedures of "*substantial severity*".[10] Applications proposing the use of wild-caught primates require "*exceptional and specific justification*". Because the potential benefit of xenotransplantation to human beings is so high the Home Office might have difficulty in refusing permission to import wild caught primates for this research. To date, however, purpose bred cynomolgus monkeys, which are readily available, have been used as primate recipients for transgenic pig kidneys.[11] Thus, it is probable that other primates, such as baboons, will not be required for this kind of research.

9 Animals (Scientific Procedures) Act 1986: Sections 5 and 7.

10 **Report of the Animal Procedures Committee for 1994** (1995) London: HMSO Cm 2996, p 7.

11 Cozzi E and White D J G (1995) The generation of transgenic pigs as potential organ donors for humans. **Nature Medicine**, 1:964-6.

5.7 Where primates are used in research as xenotransplant recipients, important welfare concerns will be raised. Because primates are highly developed they may suffer more in confinement than other animals and so the standard of care will be more critical. The Home Office sets general and worthy standards for their care and welfare.[12] In practice, however, the current standards leave much to be desired from an animal welfare viewpoint. This is demonstrated by the difference between the group housing for primates seen in good zoos and standard laboratory caging allowed under the 1986 Act.

5.8 As far as the Working Party is aware, no research intended to develop primates as sources of organs for xenografting is occurring in the UK. As set out in Chapter 4, the Working Party concluded that non-primate species should be regarded as the source animals of choice for xenotransplantation. Thus, the Working Party does not consider how far the regulatory framework does or could cover the use of primates to provide organs or tissue. If primates were to be considered as a source of organs the relevant controls would have to be reviewed.

The production and care of transgenic pigs

5.9 The process of producing transgenic pigs was summarised in Chapter 3 (paragraphs 3.27 - 3.28). Since this is a scientific procedure, which may have the effect of causing pain, suffering, distress or lasting harm to animals, it comes under the control of the 1986 Act. The 1986 Act also regulates procedures which may result in the birth of an animal that may be so affected.[13] Thus, the breeding of transgenic animals would also be covered by the 1986 Act. Transgenic vertebrates can, in principle, be released from control of the 1986 Act and used in science or agriculture, or exported to another country.[14] Release is not permitted, however, until there is satisfactory evidence that the transgene, or factors associated with transgenesis, have had no significant effect on the animal's welfare *"by the end of the normal lifespan of two generations"* [14] or *"within the lifespan of two generations"*.[15] There are two main ways in which the welfare of transgenic animals may be affected. First, the transgene itself may have a harmful effect on the animal. An example of this would be the harmful effects of genes used to make transgenic animals grow faster (paragraph 4.49). Second, the transgene may cause a harmful mutation when it is inserted into the

---

12 **Home Office Code of Practice for the Housing and Care of Animals Used in Scientific Procedures.** London: HMSO (1989). **Home Office Code of Practice for the Housing and Care of Animals in Designated Breeding and Supplying Establishments.** London: HMSO (1995).

13 Animals (Scientific Procedures) Act 1986 : Section 2.(3).

14 Home Office Policy on Transgenic Animals and "Harmful Mutants" (1994).

15 **Guide to the Genetically Modified Organisms (Contained Use) Regulations** (1992) Appendix 2; Advisory Committee on Genetic Manipulation (1989) Guidelines on Work with Transgenic Animals. ACGM/HSE Note 9, paragraphs 23-8.

genetic material of the animal. In order to be sure that this is not so, the welfare of transgenic animals must be examined in homozygous animals (those which have been bred so the transgene is present at both the possible sites in the genetic material - paragraph 3.28).

5.10 It is not clear, however, how the advice on lifespan is to be interpreted. A "*normal lifespan*", for example, may be taken to mean the normal natural lifespan, or the normal lifespan of an animal used in science or agriculture, which might be much shorter. A mouse, for example, may live as long as two years, but the average lifespan of a laboratory mouse may be nearer three months. Similarly, a pig may live for 20 - 30 years, but farmed pigs have an average lifespan of four to seven months. And "*within*" is not the same as "*by the end of*". Given these ambiguities, there is a possibility that animals may be released too early to detect a delayed effect of transgenesis on the welfare of older animals.

5.11 In addition, there may be adverse effects of transgenesis that are not detected until a relevant stimulus is encountered outside laboratory conditions. Farms, transport systems and markets, for example, are not subject to the same level of controls and monitoring as those required under the 1986 Act, and they may present transgenic animals with increased, or different, stresses.

5.12 Evidence about the suitability, or otherwise, of releasing transgenic animals from control of the 1986 Act is evaluated by the Home Office Inspectorate. Where the release of transgenic farm animals such as pigs is concerned, the Farm Animal Welfare Council will be consulted.[16] There are general criteria for assessing the welfare of these animals, but not specific criteria.[17, 18] In view of the many adverse effects that could occur from the transfer of any gene, general guidance is inevitable. It would be helpful, however, if a more precise indication was available of how animal welfare should be judged and by whom. As experience with transgenic animals increases it should be possible to develop more precise guidance for assessing their welfare.

5.13 Research into the production of transgenic farm animals is in its early stages and, to date, none have been released from the control of the 1986 Act. There is no evidence at present that the transgenic pigs developed for xenotransplantation are adversely affected by the genetic modification procedure.[19] So in principle, it is possible that,

---

16 **Report of the Animal Procedures Committee for 1990** (1991) London: HMSO Cm 1646, p 28, paragraph 7.41.

17 Home Office Policy on Transgenic Animals and "Harmful Mutants" (1994).

18 **Guide to the Genetically Modified Organisms (Contained Use) Regulations** (1992) Appendix 2; Advisory Committee on Genetic Manipulation (1989) Guidelines on Work with Transgenic Animals. ACGM/HSE Note 9, paragraphs 23-8.

19 Cozzi E and White D J G (1995) The generation of transgenic pigs as potential organ donors for humans. **Nature Medicine,** 1:964-6.

in the future, they might be released from control of the 1986 Act. Even if it is firmly established, however, that the welfare of the transgenic pigs is not affected by genetic modification, there may be other reasons not to release them from control of the 1986 Act. For example, the procedures required to produce pigs free from infectious organisms, or to remove organs and tissue may keep the pigs within control of the 1986 Act (paragraphs 5.18 - 5.26).

5.14 A slightly different situation arises if, as more animals are bred, surplus animals are generated. This is not unlikely with pigs, which can produce large litters at least twice a year, and it may become more likely if xenotransplantation were to develop into a widespread procedure. This raises the question whether such surplus animals should be made available on the general agricultural market and, in particular, whether they should be sold for human consumption. If the animals were released from the control of the 1986 Act, additional controls are in place that would regulate whether they would be made available on the general agricultural market (paragraphs 4.50 - 4.52).

5.15 If transgenic pig strains were released from control of the 1986 Act, their breeding and care, even if it were for a scientific purpose such as the treatment of human disease, would be regarded as recognised agricultural and animal husbandry practice and would not come under the control of the 1986 Act.[13, 20] As such, the welfare standards would be those pertaining to agricultural and animal husbandry practice. The Farm Animal Welfare Council advises the Ministry of Agriculture, Fisheries and Food (MAFF) on farm animal welfare. It has promoted the concept of the five freedoms, which summarise an animal's basic needs,[21] and updated the MAFF Farm Animal Welfare Codes.[22] The Farm Animal Welfare Council has expressed concern about transgenic farm animals and would oversee the welfare of any animals released from the 1986 Act.[23] Other agricultural regulations cover aspects such as notifiable diseases and transport in farm animals. Even when animals fall outside the protection of the 1986 Act, there will always be a pressure for high health standards to be maintained in the production of animals to be used for supplying organs. But there will not necessarily be the same emphasis on high welfare standards to avoid undue distress and discomfort. Inevitably, the level of monitoring and control of welfare would be reduced if animals were released from the 1986 Act.

---

20 Animals (Scientific Procedures) Act 1986 : Section 2.(8).

21 The five freedoms are: freedom from hunger and thirst, freedom from discomfort, freedom from pain, injury or disease, freedom to express normal behaviour, freedom from fear and distress.

22 MAFF **Farm Animal Welfare Codes of Recommendation for the Welfare of Livestock** made under the Agriculture (Miscellaneous Provisions) Act 1968. The Code for pigs was published in 1983 and updated by the Farm Animal Welfare Council in 1990.

23 **Report of the Animal Procedures Committee for 1990** (1991) London: HMSO Cm 1646, p 28, paragraph 7.44.

5.16 There might be a problem if two strains of transgenic pigs were interbred to produce one strain containing both transgenic modifications. Such strains might be more suitable for supplying organs for xenotransplantation (paragraph 3.32). But combining two genetic modifications might lead to welfare problems which, if the parent strains had been released from the control of the 1986 Act, might not be identified.

5.17 In addition to the controls of the 1986 Act, there are other regulations that apply to the production of transgenic organisms. The Advisory Committee on Genetic Manipulation has drawn up guidelines on work with transgenic animals.[24] The Health & Safety Executive must be informed of any research work involving the genetic modification of animals or plants.[25] The Health & Safety Executive also has to be notified of and approve the intentional release of any genetically manipulated organism into the environment. A local Genetic Manipulation Safety Committee has to advise on any risks associated with the work.[26]

The production of transgenic pigs free from infectious organisms

5.18 When considering the welfare of pigs used to provide organs or tissue for xenotransplantation, it is necessary to consider the implications of the need to breed animals that, as far as possible, are free from infectious organisms. This is important in order to reduce the risk of infectious diseases of animals passing into the human population (Chapter 6). Clearly, it will be important to produce animals that are in good health and, in this respect, they will undoubtedly be taken good care of. But there may be specific procedures that will adversely affect the welfare of the animals. In her submission to the Working Party, Hasel Prowse asked whether a transgenic pig would be able to "*roll in a field, eat ordinary pig food, mix daily with fellow pigs? Or are transgenic pigs kept in sterile conditions . . .?*"

5.19 For example, some procedures for breeding animals free from infectious organisms involve delivery by Caesarean section, after which the animals are reared in 'isolators': incubators that isolate the animal and reduce the chance of infection.[27] This would certainly have adverse effects on animal welfare. An argument against such practice is that monitoring for infectious organisms may be best carried out if

24 Advisory Committee on Genetic Manipulation (1989) Guidelines on Work with Transgenic Animals. ACGM/HSE Note 9.

25 Health & Safety at Work Act (1974); Health & Safety (Genetic Manipulation) Regulations (1978); Environmental Protection Act (1990).

26 Genetically Modified Organisms (Contained Use) Regulations (1992) (SI 1992/3217); The Genetically Modified Organisms (Deliberate Release) Regulations (1992).

27 Coates M E and Gustafsson B E eds. (1984) **The Germ-free Animal in Biomedical Research.** London. Laboratory Animals Ltd.

animals are kept in small groups. This would allow the rigorous testing of sentinel animals that have been reared with the animals from which organs or tissue will be removed.[28]

5.20 Even if isolation is not required, in order to keep animals free from infection, the environment will have to be kept relatively sterile and therefore be easy to clean. So it is likely to consist of monotonous textures and to be free of items which might enrich the life for the animal, but which might also harbour infectious organisms. Human contact, which can be advantageous for animals in captivity, may have to be minimised since human beings harbour some diseases (such as influenza) that can be passed on to pigs.

5.21 Monitoring the genetic composition of animals and screening them to make sure they are free of infectious organisms will require regular blood sampling and tissue biopsy. Invasive tests may also be required to ensure the organs and tissue to be removed are functioning properly. Even blood sampling can be quite stressful to an animal not used to such procedures. The major stress factors are the need for restraint, which may be physical and/or drug-induced, the process of removal to operating areas and the need for recovery if anaesthesia has been used. Some species can be trained for such procedures, but with pigs it is not so easy because of their size and resistance to restraint.

5.22 The need to produce animals free from infectious organisms may lead to sensory deprivation and militate against good welfare. Given some forethought, the problems are not insurmountable. Every effort must be made to reduce stress to a minimum as required by the conditions attached to a personal licence.[29] **The Working Party recommends that, when decisions are made about the acceptability of using animals for xenotransplantation, particular attention is paid to reducing the adverse effects associated with the need to produce animals free from infectious organisms.**

The removal of organs and tissue from animals

5.23 It is very likely that any company or individual will wish to administer an anaesthetic in order to remove organs or tissue from an animal. Anaesthesia is a regulated procedure under the 1986 Act[30] and, since it would be carried out on a living vertebrate for a permitted purpose, it would be subject to the controls of the 1986 Act.

---

28 A point made by David Onions in his comments to the Working Party.

29 Animals (Scientific Procedures) Act 1986 : Section 10.(2)(a).

30 Animals (Scientific Procedures) Act 1986 : Section 2.(4).

5.24 Some of the organs in the body, namely the kidneys and lungs, are paired and other organs, such as the liver, can regenerate. Other structures, such as the pancreatic islets and the skin, may contain sufficient tissue for transplantation into more than one patient. Thus it would be possible, in principle, to remove tissue and organs sequentially from an animal until a vital organ was removed: either the heart or the second kidney. The sequential removal of organs or tissues in this way would involve repeated restraint, anaesthesia and recovery and could give rise to unnecessary suffering. This raises the issue of the regulation of the repeated use of animals under the 1986 Act.

5.25 Subjecting animals to multiple procedures is carefully regulated by the 1986 Act. Taking a biopsy to ensure the suitability of an organ or tissue, even if that required giving the animal a general anaesthetic, would not preclude the subsequent removal of the organs from the animal. Sequential removal of organs or tissue, however, when another animal could equally well be used, would be classified as re-use. The Home Office have stated that such re-use would be prohibited because the use of another animal would cause less suffering.[31] **The Working Party recommends that the Animals (Scientific Procedures) Act 1986 should continue to be interpreted as prohibiting sequential removal from animals of tissues or organs for transplantation.**

5.26 What if animals were to be killed, and the organs removed, without the use of an anaesthetic? Killing animals is normally subject only to the standards of recognised agricultural or animal husbandry practice. Even for animals whose use is regulated under the 1986 Act, killing the animals may not be regulated.[32] It is worth noting that slaughtermen now have to be trained and licensed. Any concern revolving around the humaneness of the methods used to kill animals for xenotransplantation would have to be brought within the scope of the Protection of Animals Act 1911 (in Scotland, the 1912 Act). Someone may be prosecuted under the 1911 Act if it can be proved an animal has been caused "*unnecessary suffering*". A court would have to decide, for any action, whether the "*procedures*" involved caused "*unnecessary suffering.*" It has been notoriously difficult to obtain a conviction on this charge in the past.[33] One of the specific aims of the Royal Society for the Prevention of Cruelty to Animals is to ensure that "*killing of animals [reared for production of cells and tissues] is humane and that it is only carried out by people with appropriate training.*"[34]

---

31 Animals (Scientific Procedures) Act 1986 : Section 10.(2)(a).

32 "*Killing a protected animal is a regulated procedure only if it is killed for experimental or other scientific use, the place where it is killed is a designated establishment and the method employed is not one appropriate to the animal under Schedule 1 to this Act.*" Animals (Scientific Procedures) Act 1986 : Section 2.(7).

33 Protection of Animals Act (1911, 1912 Scotland).

34 A position set out in the RSPCA's submission to the Working Party.

Conclusion

5.27 This chapter has set out the welfare implications of: breeding transgenic animals; producing animals free, as far as possible, from infectious organisms; and removing organs and tissue from animals for xenotransplantation. There is some uncertainty about whether, in practice, all these aspects would be covered by the 1986 Act. In view of the important welfare implications raised by xenotransplantation, **the Working Party recommends that the Home Office should require that all animals used for xenotransplantation are protected under the Animals (Scientific Procedures) Act 1986.** Any reputable company producing animals in order to supply organs and tissue for xenotransplantation would, in any case, wish to be licensed under the 1986 Act in order to reassure the public that their activities were meeting the highest standards of animal welfare. **The Working Party recommends that the standards set by the 1986 Act become the minimum for the industry.**

Chapter 6

Transmission of infectious diseases

6.1 In principle, xenografts, if successful, would offer huge benefits to individual patients. Xenografting, however, may also involve certain risks. This chapter discusses the risk that using animals to supply organs will result in the transmission of infectious diseases from animals to the human population. As discussed in Chapter 4, the Working Party recommends that the development of xenotransplantation should involve pigs, not primates as source animals (paragraph 4.40). One important reason contributing to that decision is the greater concern about disease transmission from primates. The evidence for that concern is presented in this chapter. The fact that xenotransplantation of baboon organs and tissue into human beings is proposed and, indeed, already occurring in the US[1] is a further reason for discussing the risks that diseases will pass from primates to xenograft recipients and thereby into the wider population.

6.2 Many disease-causing organisms (pathogens) are common to human beings and other animals.[2] For example, the bacterium causing tuberculosis infects both human beings and baboons, and human beings and pigs both carry the virus that causes influenza. Clearly it would be important to make sure that any animal used to supply organs was free from infectious organisms that cause disease in human beings, just as it is important to make sure that human organ donors are free from infections that might be transmitted to a transplant recipient. The use of animals as a source of organs, it is argued, would allow for more thorough screening than is possible with human organ donors, and so the risk of such diseases might be reduced.

6.3 In addition to organisms that can infect both human beings and other animals, any animal species will be infected with organisms that do not usually infect other species. Xenotransplantation, however, may allow such organisms to infect xenograft recipients who may, consequently, contract previously unknown diseases. There is also a risk that the infectious organisms might cause disease in and destroy the transplanted organ, even if they do not harm the human recipient. Even if not infected with disease-causing organisms when transplanted, the xenografted organ may remain susceptible to infectious organisms of animals. This is most likely to be a problem with lung transplants, where infectious organisms of animals would easily get access to the transplanted animal tissue. Any person thinking about volunteering

1 Aids patient given baboon bone marrow. (1995) **Lancet**, 378:756.

2 The word 'organisms' should be taken to include viruses and prions. While not strictly correct, the Working Party adopted this convention in the interests of accessibility and brevity.

for a xenograft would have to be made aware of, and to consider these risks, about which very little is known at present, along with all the other factors that would need to be taken into account (paragraphs 7.14 - 7.21).

6.4 The possibility must also be considered that should an animal organism infect a xenograft recipient the resultant disease might then be passed on to the public at large. In this way, xenografting may pose a risk to public health as well as to individual health. Many of those who responded to the public consultation emphasised the importance of addressing the risks of disease transmission associated with xenotransplantation.[3] This chapter considers, first, the possibility that new diseases will be transmitted from animals to xenograft recipients. It then considers the risks that such diseases might spread from xenograft recipients into the general population. Finally, the principles by which these risks might be assessed and managed are discussed.

The risk that infectious organisms will be transmitted from animals to human beings

6.5 There is evidence that human beings are susceptible to some animal diseases. Such diseases are called zoonoses. For example:

- human beings in contact with monkeys can become infected with monkeypox virus, which is related to the smallpox virus;
- contact with macaque monkeys can lead to infection with a macaque form of herpes B virus which causes encephalitis in human beings which is rapidly fatal;
- the human immunodeficiency virus (HIV) virus that causes AIDS is very similar to the simian immunodeficiency viruses (SIV) found in primates. One view attributes the emergence of the HIV virus and the disease AIDS in human beings to the transmission of SIV viruses from primates to human beings. There is evidence that the SIV virus can, indeed, be transmitted from primates to human beings although, as yet, there is no evidence of disease symptoms in SIV infected human beings.[4, 5]

3 These included Animal Aid, the British Union for the Abolition of Vivisection, the Christian Medical Fellowship, the Church of England, the Church of Scotland, the Church in Wales, Professor David Onions, the Genetics Forum, the Jain Academy, Professor John Polkinghorne and PPL Therapeutics.

4 Chapman L E *et al.* (1995) Xenotransplantation and xenogeneic infections. **New England Journal of Medicine**, 333:1498-501.

5 Thanks, but no thanks. **The Economist**, 21 October 1995, pp 17, 137-9.

6.6 Xenotransplantation is one way by which disease-causing organisms could be transferred from animals to human beings. Because xenotransplantation involves the direct introduction of animal organs or tissue into the human body, many of the natural barriers to infection are by-passed. Xenograft recipients are also likely to require immunosuppression to prevent transplant rejection. Since immunosuppression lowers the body's resistance to disease, the possibility of infection of a recipient with animal diseases may be increased further.

6.7 It is sometimes argued that the risk of transmission of animal diseases is overestimated, since immunosuppressed recipients of human organ transplants who are in contact with pets or farm animals, do not contract animal diseases. This argument, however, ignores the major difference between close contact with animals and the transfer of animal organs or tissue directly into the human body. The potential importance of this difference is illustrated by the following example. Cats are susceptible to infection by feline leukaemia virus. Dogs or human beings, in contact with cats, do not become infected with the virus. But if young, immunosuppressed dogs are transplanted with infected cat tissue, the dogs become infected with the virus and develop tumours.[6]

Infectious organisms

6.8 Xenografting provides a potential route for the transmission of disease. So it is necessary to consider the organisms that infect possible source animals and to assess whether they are likely to cause disease in human beings. Important categories of infectious organisms include viruses, bacteria and fungi. Prion proteins are another type of infectious agent that are thought to cause diseases such as bovine spongiform encephalopathy (BSE, or 'mad cow disease') and human Creutzfeldt-Jakob Disease (CJD). There is evidence that prion diseases can pass from one species to another.[7] Thus, prion disease transmission is another risk that needs to be considered when contemplating xenografting.

6.9 Most concern about the risks of infection from xenotransplantation focuses on viruses. This is because:

1 viral infections are difficult to treat with drugs;

2 viral infections may have a long latent period during which the person has no symptoms of the disease. This is the case with HIV infection: it may take 10 years for an infected person to develop AIDS. If a new disease were to

6 Onions D (1995) Comments made at an Institute of Medicine conference on Xenograft transplantation: science, ethics and public policy, Washington DC.

7 Prusiner S (1995) The prion diseases. **Scientific American**, 272(1):30-7.

emerge as a consequence of xenotransplantation, it might be several years before the problem was identified. During this time the infection might be spreading throughout the population;

3 viruses can mutate rapidly and thereby change their characteristics.[8] Mutation might allow animal viruses to infect human beings more readily; to resist attack by the human immune system; or to become drug-resistant;

4 one type of mutation occurs when viruses from different species recombine with each other and form new and possibly more dangerous viruses. It is thought that influenza epidemics are caused when new types of influenza virus are formed by recombination of two viruses, sometimes from different species. Xenotransplantation would provide increased opportunities for recombination between animal and human viruses;

5 one group of viruses, known as endogenous retroviruses, are inserted into the genetic material of the host animal and can be passed in this way from parent to offspring. This makes endogenous retroviruses almost impossible to eliminate from any animals that might be used as a source of organs for xenografting. It is possible that, after xenotransplantation, the endogenous retroviruses would move from the transplanted organs and become inserted into the genetic material of the human cells. Such insertion may cause mutations in the human genetic material and lead to an increased risk of cancer.[9]

Comparison of the risks to human beings from infectious organisms of primates and pigs

6.10 The high degree of genetic relatedness of human beings and other primates means that infectious organisms from primates may have a good chance of surviving in, and causing disease in, human beings. Baboons, for example, carry several viruses with the potential to infect human beings including several herpes viruses (SA8, simian cytomegalovirus, and herpes papio) and several retroviruses (STLV-1, baboon endogenous retrovirus and foamy virus).[10] As mentioned above, there is considerable evidence that primates do indeed carry viruses that infect and cause disease in human beings (paragraph 6.5). These risks are reflected in the safety

8 This is especially likely for RNA viruses, including retroviruses, which replicate less faithfully than DNA viruses.

9 Stoye J P and Coffin J M (1995) The dangers of xenotransplantation. Letter to **Nature Medicine,** 1:1100.

10 Allan J S (1995) Xenotransplantation at a crossroads: Prevention versus progress. **Nature Medicine,** 2:18-21.

precautions taken by people handling primates.[11] There is also experimental evidence that endogenous retroviruses from baboons can infect human cells.[12] Because the viruses from human beings and other primates are often closely related, the risk of recombination to form new harmful viruses, may be high (paragraph 6.9.4). Another problem is that to breed primates free from known viruses, in so far as this is possible, would require a long-term programme because of their relatively slow breeding rates (paragraph 4.34). As discussed below, there are certain to be primate viruses that are currently unidentified and which may have the potential to cause disease in human beings (paragraph 6.14).

6.11 In contrast, the more marked biological differences between pigs and human beings, and between their infectious organisms, may make it more difficult for infectious organisms from pigs to cause disease in human beings. Moreover, pigs have been domesticated and used by human beings for centuries, yet there is no evidence for transmission of viral diseases into the human population on the scale seen with viral diseases of other primates. Although the risks are likely to be lower, however, they cannot be ignored. Imutran Ltd, the UK firm developing transgenic pigs for xenotransplantation have pointed out that "*the particular concern that xenografting raises is the risk of transmitting a pig pathogen to a human.*"[13] Pig viruses with the potential to infect human beings include those causing porcine influenza, parainfluenza, swine vesicular disease, encephalomyocarditis and, possibly, pseudorabies.[14] Pigs, like primates, contain endogenous retroviruses and studies are needed to assess whether they can infect human cells.[15] Since they have a shorter generation time than primates, breeding pigs free of known viruses should prove more feasible. Pigs, however, will also contain viruses and other infectious organisms that have not yet been identified. Moreover, at least initially, recipients of pig xenografts might require high levels of immunosuppression which would render them very susceptible to infections. However, the hope is that, eventually, relatively low levels of immunosuppression could be used if organs are taken from transgenic pigs that have been genetically modified to reduce the immune response after transplantation.[16]

---

11 Whitney R A and Wickings E J (1987) Macaques and other old world simians, Chapter 40 of **The UFAW Handbook on the Care and Management of Laboratory Animals** Sixth Edition. UK: Longman Scientific & Technical.

12 Benveniste R *et al.* (1974) Infectious type-C virus isolated from baboon placenta. **Nature** (London), 248:17-20.

13 Imutran Ltd: submission to the Working Party.

14 Onions D: submission to the Working Party.

15 Stoye J P and Coffin J M (1995) The dangers of xenotransplantation. Letter to **Nature Medicine,** 1:1100.

16 Cozzi E and White D J G (1995) The generation of transgenic pigs as potential organ donors for humans. **Nature Medicine,** 1:964-6.

6.12 The evidence suggests that the risk of disease transmission from primates will be greater than that from pigs. This conclusion supports the Working Party's recommendation that non-primate species should be regarded as the source animals of choice for xenotransplantation. Nevertheless, the risks of disease transmission from pigs also need careful consideration. It is sometimes argued that pig heart valves have been transplanted into human beings for more than 30 years without any evidence of disease transmission. Pig heart valves, however, are fixed in glutaraldehyde, a process that renders them non-viable and which would reduce, if not eliminate, all infectious organisms.[17] This treatment would not be possible for organs and tissue that are to be transplanted whilst still viable.

Assessing the risks of infection

6.13 It is important to know as much as possible about the infectious organisms present in the animal species that are most likely to be developed as sources for xenografts, namely baboons and pigs. It is, however, very difficult to determine whether organisms that cause disease in animals will also infect and cause disease in human beings. Another difficulty is that it is not uncommon for infectious organisms, that are harmless or cause relatively mild symptoms in their natural host, to cause more severe disease in a different species. One example is macaque herpes B virus which causes severe human encephalitis in human beings (paragraph 6.5).

6.14 Another problem is that there are undoubtedly infectious organisms of both primates and pigs that are currently unknown. This is true even of human beings: in the last few years, three new herpes viruses have been identified (herpes viruses 6, 7 and 8).[18] It will be very difficult to identify organisms that do not cause any symptoms in the animal from which they come. Previous experience indicates that infectious organisms are normally identified only after the emergence of the disease they cause. The HIV virus, for example, was only identified after the emergence of the disease AIDS. Put bluntly, it may be possible to identify any infectious organism transmitted by xenografting only if it causes disease in human beings, and after it has started to do so. Even this may be difficult if, as with AIDS, there is a long latent period between infection and development of the disease. Animal Aid pointed out in their submission that "*cross species transplants carry a further, potentially devastating risk in that a currently unknown (and therefore unscreened for) animal virus could trigger a new plague when it crossed the species barrier.*"

---

17 Marks C and Marks P (1993) **Fundamentals of cardiac surgery.** London: Chapman & Hall Medical, pp 105-9.

18 Herpes virus 6: Salahuddin S *et al.* (1986) Isolation of a new virus, HBLV, in patients with lymphoproliferative disorders. **Science,** 234:596-601. Herpes virus 7: Frenkel N *et al.* (1990) Isolation of a new herpesvirus from human CD4+ T-cells. **Proceedings of the National Academy of Sciences, USA,** 87:748-52. Herpes virus 8: Chang Y *et al.* (1994) Identification of herpesvirus-like DNA sequences in AIDS-associated Kaposi's sarcoma. **Science,** 266:1865-9.

6.15 Just as with any other medical advance, it is impossible to eliminate all risk or, even, to be able to predict and quantify all the risks associated with xenotransplantation. But it is important to make a clear distinction between the unquantifiable risks and the risks that can be usefully investigated. It is necessary to be sure that all the research that can usefully be done has been completed before clinical trials involving human beings are contemplated. A variety of experimental approaches will help identify, quantify and eliminate some of the risks of infection associated with xenografting (paragraphs 6.24 - 6.26).

The risk of animal diseases spreading from xenograft recipients into the general population

6.16 While some infectious organisms of animals may cause disease if they are transferred directly into a xenograft recipient, they may not be able to pass from person to person. Infectious organisms may need to change their characteristics before they can spread into the human population. It is known that disease-causing organisms of one animal species can undergo changes enabling them to infect different animals. One example is the feline parvovirus, that has infected at least two new hosts, mink and dogs, in the last 40 years.[19] On the whole, however, changes of this kind are more likely to occur within a large number of organisms, that is, amongst the organisms found in the animals they normally infect. Such changes are less likely to arise within the small number of organisms that would be found in xenograft recipients. An exception to this would be the retroviruses since xenotransplantation would increase the risk of recombination between animal and human viruses (paragraph 6.9.4). This might produce a new virus that was able to pass efficiently from human being to human being. Conversely, prion diseases are unlikely to pass into the wider population, even if they infect individual recipients (paragraph 6.8). This is because transmission of prion diseases is normally by transplantation or by eating infected material.

6.17 It is extremely difficult to assess the level of risk that an animal disease will be transmitted to the human population as a result of xenotransplantation. Experts in the field vary widely in their opinions.[20] The conclusion would seem to be that, when considering the possibility of xenografting leading to the transmission of disease into the human population, the risk is unquantifiable and it may be extremely small. But it cannot be ruled out.

19 Parrish C (1990) Emergence, natural history, and variation of canine, mink and feline parvoviruses. **Advances in Virus Research**, 38:404-50.

20 Allan J S (1995) Xenotransplantation at a crossroads: Prevention versus progress. **Nature Medicine**, 2:18-21.

6.18 Someone who required a life-saving operation would probably be prepared to accept a risk of infection which is greater than that thought to be acceptable for the whole population. The ethical question is how to balance the needs of individual transplant recipients, and the potential benefits to them of xenotransplantation, against the uncertainties associated with the possible transmission of a new infectious disease to the general population. Even allowing that xenografts might bring benefits to patients in terms of increased quality and length of life, the potential public health risks nevertheless counsel caution. The consent of individuals to take these risks does not justify their imposition upon the public.

6.19 In other areas of medical and scientific developments, it has been found appropriate to limit the associated risks by establishing regulatory mechanisms. Examples are the regulations controlling the development of new medicines, and of gene therapy techniques. Where there is a perceived risk to public health, or the environment, there is further increased rigour, as seen in the area of genetically modified organisms (paragraphs 4.50 - 4.52). This suggests the urgent need in the field of xenografting to establish agreement on best practice and the appropriate regulation of xenografting procedures.

The principle of precaution

6.20 As set out above, the development of xenotransplantation is associated with the potential risk of transmission of new diseases to the human population. It is not possible to predict or quantify this risk but, in the worst case, the consequences could be far-reaching and difficult to control. In this type of situation, a cost/benefit approach to dealing with risk analysis has limitations because the costs (and, indeed, the benefits) are not known and cannot be predicted. Since the possible consequences of developing xenotransplantation are potentially very serious, it is hardly wise to use a method of risk analysis that cannot address such consequences until they start to be seen.

6.21 The principle of precaution offers an alternative method of risk analysis and assessment.[21] This has been developed within the field of environmental policy and applied to the control of pollution and the release of genetically modified organisms. The principle of precaution requires that action should be taken to avoid risks **in advance of** certainty about their nature. This challenges the view that, until there is evidence that a new technology is harmful, it is acceptable to proceed with its development. It suggests that the burden of proof should lie with those developing the technology to demonstrate that it will not cause serious harm.

---

21 O'Riordan T and Jordan A (1995) The Precautionary Principle in Contemporary Environmental Politics. **Environmental Values**, 4:191-212.

6.22 An implication of the principle of precaution is that the development of some technologies simply should not be pursued. Since any innovation must by definition carry some unknowable risks, however, it would be unacceptably conservative to restrict innovation merely by appeal to the possibility of risk. For each technology, an attempt must be made to identify and define the risks and to decide on a course of action. It may be that, for some technologies, the principle of precaution would argue that they should not be pursued. For others, it will be possible to identify safeguards that will reduce the risks of the technology.

6.23 What are the implications of the principle of precaution when applied to the uncertainties associated with disease transmission via xenotransplantation? The discussion above has set out the potential risk from infectious organisms of animals and highlighted the difficulties in identifying these organisms, determining whether they will cause disease in human beings and predicting whether the diseases will spread to the wider population. **The Working Party concluded that the risks associated with possible transmission of infectious diseases as a consequence of xenotransplantation have not been adequately dealt with. It would not be ethical, therefore to begin clinical trials of xenotransplantation involving human beings.** In order to address the risks of disease transmission associated with xenotransplantation, the Working Party suggests that the following measures should be taken:

- stringent efforts should be made to assemble as much information as possible about the risks of disease transmission **before** further xenotransplantation goes ahead. This would involve reviewing existing research and undertaking new research where necessary on the infectious organisms of primates and pigs and the possibility of transmission of disease to human beings (paragraphs 6.24 - 6.26);
- xenotransplantation should use only source animals reared in conditions in which all known infectious organisms are monitored and controlled. It is ethically unacceptable to use source organs from animals that are known to be infected with infectious organisms that can be eliminated (paragraphs 6.27 - 6.32);
- there should be thorough monitoring of early recipients, with regular testing for signs and symptoms of disease (paragraphs 6.33 - 6.37);
- there should be a commitment to suspend, modify or, if necessary, discontinue xenotransplantation procedures at any signs that new infectious diseases are emerging.

The next sections discuss these requirements in more detail.

Assembling information about the risks of disease transmission

6.24 Experimental studies can be used to try to identify unknown infectious agents in animal tissue.[22] Transplantation of pig or baboon tissue into immunocompromised mice might allow the identification of previously unknown infectious organisms. It is also possible to test whether animal viruses will infect human cells grown in the laboratory, using co-cultivation techniques in which human cells and infected animal cells are grown in the same container. This technique has shown that baboon retroviruses can infect human cells. New molecular techniques allow virologists to search for the genetic material of previously unknown viruses.[23]

6.25 Such research is not without its difficulties. Results obtained using human cells in tissue culture may not always be applicable to human recipients. But there is no doubt that much useful laboratory research can be done, particularly in the area of endogenous retroviruses which may present particular risks. Useful research could be done to identify the different retroviruses present in source animals, to assess whether the viruses are activated by transplantation, and to examine the rate of mutation shown by the viruses. Research involving animal xenograft recipients could be useful in this respect. Primate recipients of pig organs, for example, could be assessed in order to determine whether porcine retroviruses are activated after transplantation, and whether the viruses then infect the primate tissue.

6.26 Another area where research is needed is in improving the diagnostic tests used to identify infectious organisms. Many of the tests used to identify infectious organisms in animals were originally developed as tests for closely related organisms that infect human beings. When the tests are used with animals, the results are often less reliable, increasing the risk that an animal with a negative test result may in fact be infected with the organism. The technology is now available to develop tests which analyse the genetic material of infectious organisms. Such DNA-based analysis is often more reliable than tests which measure the antibody levels in the human or animal. Antibody tests have the drawback that they do not work well in patients who are immunosuppressed and therefore have low levels of antibody. Reliable, accurate and more sensitive methods of diagnosing infection in animals and human beings should be available and regularly used before clinical xenotransplantation trials go ahead.

---

22 Onions D and Lees G, Human herpesviruses and retroviruses: problems and solutions in the safety testing of biologicals in Horaud F and Brown F eds. (1990) **Developments in Biological Standardisation**, 75:145-158.

23 Representational difference analysis, for example, basically involves comparing the genetic material of uninfected organisms with that of potentially infected organisms: any extra material may be due to the presence of an infectious organism (Lisitsyn N *et al.* (1993) Cloning the difference between two complex genomes. **Science**, 259:946-51). Organisms can also be identified using polymerase chain reaction techniques with primers based on the sequence of organisms potentially related to the unknown organism (Compton T, Degenerate primers for DNA amplification. Chapter in Innis M A *et al.* eds. (1990) **PCR Protocols: A guide to methods and applications.** Academic Press).

Producing animals free from known infectious organisms

6.27 Because of the potential dangers of disease transmission, xenotransplant teams have sought to produce source animals free from known infectious organisms. The animals are reared in captivity and maintained in a clean environment. Individual animals are tested regularly to check levels of infection. Precautions are also taken to ensure that human beings rearing the animals do not inadvertently infect them with human diseases, such as influenza. In order to eliminate other viruses, a long-term breeding programme and intensive screening would be required. This would be a particularly lengthy process for primates.[24] In addition, it might be necessary to use methods such as delivery of animals by Caesarean section, and rearing of animals in isolation. This would have implications for the welfare of the animals (Chapter 5). Moreover, it is essentially impossible to eliminate retroviruses that have become inserted into the genetic material of the host animal (paragraph 6.9.5).

6.28 There is currently no general agreement amongst xenograft teams as to precisely which organisms should be excluded from animal sources. Thus, some xenografts have already taken place which have used animals infected with known organisms. For example, the baboons used as sources for the two liver xenotransplant recipients in Pittsburgh were known to be infected with foamy virus, a member of the retrovirus family.[25] Neither patient showed evidence of foamy virus infection during the short time they lived after their operations. Baboon foamy virus is not known to infect human beings, but some foamy viruses have the ability to infect several species. For example, some mouse foamy viruses can infect human cells. While there is no evidence to date that foamy viruses cause diseases in their hosts, some virologists nevertheless hold the view that foamy viruses should be eliminated from animals used to provide xenografts.[26]

6.29 The term **specified-pathogen free** is used to describe animals from which specified infectious organisms (pathogens) have been excluded. But, as the example above makes clear, there is no consensus about which organisms should be excluded from specified-pathogen free animals. **The Working Party recommends that a code of practice should be drawn up specifying which organisms should be excluded from specified-pathogen free animals. Xenotransplantation teams should be required to exclude from source animals all the pathogens listed in the code of practice.** Mechanisms should be in place to allow the list of organisms to be updated in the light of experience. The code of practice should recommend the diagnostic tests to be performed by accredited test centres.

---

24 Allan J S (1995) Xenotransplantation at a crossroads: Prevention versus progress. **Nature Medicine**, 2:18-21.

25 Michaels M (1995) Presentation at an Institute of Medicine conference on Xenograft transplantation: science, ethics and public policy, Washington DC.

26 Allan J (1995) Xenotransplantation and the infectious disease conundrum. **Institute of Laboratory Animal Resources Journal**, 37:37-48; Onions D (1995) Comments made at an Institute of Medicine conference on Xenograft transplantation: science, ethics and public policy, Washington DC.

6.30 It must be borne in mind that specified-pathogen free status can apply only to known infectious organisms. Specified-pathogen free animals may still be infected with unidentified infectious organisms about which nothing is known (paragraph 6.14).

6.31 In addition to the elimination of pathogens from the whole animal, it may also be necessary to perform tests on the organ or tissue intended for xenotransplantation to ensure that it is free from infectious organisms and, more generally, that it is of a high quality. In the case of transgenic pigs, for example, it will be necessary to ensure that the organ or tissue does indeed carry the correct genetic modification.

6.32 A regulatory framework will be needed to ensure the quality and safety of xenografts. How far would current regulations cover xenografts? The Medical Devices Directive regulates the use of some, but not all, products used for medical treatment. The Directive excludes "*transplants or tissues or cells of animal origin, unless a device is manufactured utilizing animal tissue which is rendered non-viable or non-viable products derived from animal tissue.*" [27] Since most animal organs and tissue used for xenotransplantation will be viable, they will be excluded from the Directive. Human organs and tissue are also excluded from the Directive.[28] A previous report of the Nuffield Council on Bioethics has highlighted the lack of a coherent regulatory structure for controlling the quality and safety of human organs and tissue.[29] This means that there is no regulatory mechanism which could be adapted for animal organs and tissue. **The Working Party recommends that a regulatory framework is devised to control the safety and quality of animal organs and tissue for xenotransplantation.** Such regulation should require the development of protocols describing the production of organs and documentation of the production process. This would enable every stage of the production of an individual organ to be controlled and checked, from preparation of the DNA required for production of the transgenic animal to screening of the source animal and transplantation of the organ. The protocols should include archiving of serum and/or tissue samples from the source animal.

Follow-up of xenograft recipients

6.33 There is a need for thorough monitoring and surveillance of early recipients of xenografts. As described earlier, a number of xenografts involving human beings have already taken place (Table 3.1). In some cases, the life of the recipient did not

27 Council Directive 93/42/EEC of 14 June concerning medical devices, Article 1.5(g). **Official Journal of the European Communities, L 169**, Vol 36, 12 July 1993.

28 Council Directive 93/42/EEC of 14 June concerning medical devices, Article 1.5(f). **Official Journal of the European Communities, L 169**, Vol 36, 12 July 1993.

29 Nuffield council on Bioethics (1995) Safety and Quality, Chapter 12 in **Human Tissue: Ethical and Legal Issues.**

depend on the success of the transplant. Thus, in one study, fetal pig pancreatic islets were transplanted into eight diabetic patients.[30] The surviving recipients of these, and other, xenografts represent good subjects for further follow-up in order to assess whether there has been any transmission of infection from the source animal to the recipient.

6.34 It is equally important to establish procedures for monitoring any future recipients of xenografts. What level of monitoring and follow-up would ensure that any signs of infectious disease are picked up early, but at the same time would not constitute too much of an imposition? It is possible to highlight a number of important features of any follow-up. Regular physical examinations with archiving of serum and, where appropriate, tissue samples should continue throughout the lifetime of the recipient. Serum samples taken from health care workers caring for the xenograft recipients should also be archived. The recipient should be required to report any serious unexplained illness. Close contacts, that is, family members, household members, sexual contacts and others with whom bodily fluids may be shared, should also be encouraged to report unexplained illnesses. Recipients should be asked to agree to an autopsy on their death.

6.35 In addition, xenograft recipients should be asked to take routine precautions to minimise the transmission of any infectious disease. They should not donate blood, tissue or organs. They should be counselled on methods of minimising the transmission of diseases, for example, by sexual contact.

6.36 The most difficult question is what procedures should be followed if it is found that a disease has indeed been transmitted from the animals used to provide organs or tissue to human xenograft recipients? In principle, steps should be taken to prevent transmission of the disease to other people. In practice, this is a very difficult issue. For a start, it is very unlikely that, at the outset, the mode of transmission of the disease will be understood. The appropriate response will depend on the mode of transmission and on how infectious the disease is. It would hardly be acceptable to isolate xenograft recipients suffering from an infectious disease, or to ask them to refrain from sexual intercourse or, in the case of a virus transmitted from parent to offspring, from having children. This highlights how difficult it would be to prevent the transmission of an infectious disease originating from xenotransplantation. It is sobering to reflect on the difficulty, despite globally coordinated attempts, of controlling and eliminating infectious diseases such as malaria, hepatitis and AIDS. This demonstrates the importance of taking steps to reduce as far as possible the risk that a new disease will emerge before trials involving human beings take place. **The Working Party recommends that standards and mechanisms for monitoring xenograft recipients and for the action to be taken in case of disease transmission should be in place before human trials begin. It should be a requirement of**

30 Groth C G *et al.* (1994) Transplantation of porcine fetal pancreas to diabetic patients. **Lancet,** 344:1402-4.

clinical trials that the need for monitoring is explained to the patient and that it is made clear that consent to the operation also implies consent to subsequent monitoring.

6.37 In order to facilitate the recording and analysis of information concerning possible disease transmission, **the Working Party recommends that xenotransplantation teams should be required to record all information concerning individual xenograft recipients in a xenotransplantation register maintained by an independent body.** Suitably anonymised data should be reviewed for evidence of the possible emergence of new diseases. Since, initially, xenograft recipients are likely to be few, and to be spread across several countries, international co-operation should take place to enable effective review of all the available evidence.

Conclusion

6.38 Xenotransplantation of animal organs and tissue carries with it the potential risk of transmission of disease to xenograft recipients and to the wider human population. Since the possible consequences of developing xenotransplantation are potentially very serious, the principle of precaution should apply. This requires that action is taken to avoid risks in advance of certainty about their nature. This chapter has set out what action would be required by the serious application of the principle of precaution to the development of xenotransplantation. To arrive at the necessary consensus about good practice, and the mechanisms to ensure that such good practice is adhered to, a body of expertise, of authority and of independence from the research teams at work on xenotransplantation is required. In view of the seriousness of the issues and of the public concerns about the technique, **the Working Party recommends that the Department of Health should establish an Advisory Committee on Xenotransplantation.**

6.39 One possible model for the proposed Advisory Committee on Xenotransplantation is the Gene Therapy Advisory Committee (GTAC). GTAC is a non-statutory Committee that was established in 1993 to "*consider and advise on the acceptability of proposals for gene therapy research on human subjects*".[31] Like GTAC, the proposed Advisory Committee on Xenotransplantation should combine the necessary scientific and medical expertise to examine early protocols with broader expertise to ensure that the Committee keeps in mind the wide range of issues raised by xenotransplantation. The proposed Committee should be open and accountable: qualities valued by many of those who made submissions to the Working Party. The Methodist Church wrote: *"the management and oversight of [xenotransplantation] can best be achieved through a regulatory and licensing body which is also charged with the*

31 Gene Therapy Advisory Committee (March 1995) **First Annual Report November 1993-December 1994**, Health Departments of the United Kingdom. p 6.

task of examining the ethical dimensions of xenografts in the light of structured public discussion."

6.40 The Working Party accepts that there will be reluctance to create another Advisory Committee. But the UK Government has a good record in establishing stringent controls to monitor developments in genetic engineering. It has been possible to reduce these controls where developments have proved satisfactory over a term of years.

6.41 **The Working Party recommends that the proposed Advisory Committee on Xenotransplantation should produce guidance on best practice and revise that guidance in the light of experience. The responsibilities of the Advisory Committee should include:**

- **assembling and assessing information about the possible risks of disease transmission and, on that basis, making recommendations (paragraphs 6.24 - 6.26);**
- **establishing a regulatory mechanism to ensure that the appropriate infectious organisms are eliminated from source animals (paragraphs 6.27 - 6.32); and**
- **developing guidance on the monitoring of future recipients of xenografts and maintaining a register of xenograft recipients (paragraph 6.33 - 6.37).**

No xenotransplantation trials involving human recipients should proceed until the proposed Advisory Committee on Xenotransplantation is in place and the above issues have been addressed.

6.42 Animals used for xenotransplantation, the Working Party has recommended, should be protected by a system whereby the Animal Procedures Committee examines all applications to use animals for this purpose (paragraph 5.5). There will be a need for close liaison between the proposed Advisory Committee on Xenotransplantation and the Animal Procedures Committee. The Advisory Committee will be in a position to advise the Animal Procedures Committee on the expected benefits of xenotransplantation which would need to be weighed against the harm to the animals. The Animal Procedures Committee will be able to advise the Advisory Committee on the welfare implications of measures to eliminate infectious organisms from source animals.

Chapter 7

Early patients

7.1 Many important medical innovations have not been immediately successful. This may well be true for xenotransplantation. This raises two major questions:

- at what stage will it be ethical to progress from using animals as xenograft recipients to the first clinical trials involving human recipients of xenografts?
- how can the welfare of the first patients to undergo xenotransplantation be protected? If it is ethical in principle for them to be offered xenotransplantation as an experimental treatment, what safeguards are needed to ensure that their consent to participation is given freely and with adequate understanding of what will be involved?

When will xenotransplantation trials involving human beings be justified?

7.2 As discussed in Chapter 3, there are significant scientific hurdles to be overcome before xenotransplantation can be clinically successful. Progress has been made in controlling the rejection of xenografts by the immune system, as indicated by the increasing lengths of time that xenografted organs or tissue survive when transplanted into animals used as experimental recipients (paragraph 3.29). The question is: at what point will the results from experiments using animals as recipients justify clinical trials involving human beings?

7.3 Experience with other major developments in medicine, such as human organ transplantation, the use of mechanical organs and, indeed, the few xenotransplants already performed, suggest that early xenograft recipients will not have a good chance of survival (Table 3.1). To an extent this is inevitable since, by their nature, trials of new treatments involve unknown and unpredictable risks. It will be impossible to predict, for example, whether a pig kidney will function properly in a human body, until the first transplants into human beings are performed. Thus, even when the results from animal experiments suggest that xenotransplantation involving human beings is justifiable, these will be major and risky operations. Because of this, it is important not to perform xenotransplants on human recipients prematurely. Advocates of early clinical trials of xenotransplantation point to the desperate situation of patients waiting for human organs for transplantation, many of whom will die before suitable organs become available. It is certainly crucial to ensure that no unnecessary obstacles are put in the way of treating these patients. But it should also be remembered that the first heart transplant, performed by Christian Barnard in South Africa in 1967, was followed by a worldwide spate of unsuccessful attempts to perform heart transplants. The reaction to these operations, which were seen as ill-judged and premature, slowed the subsequent development of successful heart transplantation. This disadvantaged the group of patients that it had been intended to benefit.

7.4 While recognising that medicine has made huge strides as a result of experimentation, members of the Working Party felt that these had sometimes been achieved at the expense of the first patients to be given the new treatment. These first patients might sometimes have been better served by an approach more accepting of death: an approach that preserved dignity and reduced suffering to a minimum. In some cases, it has been cruel to offer a possible life-saving procedure that resulted in a long drawn-out, painful death, instead of a relatively peaceful end. The offer of such a procedure in itself puts pressure on patients to accept - and may distort judgement.

7.5 Yet there will be many patients for whom the chance of making a contribution to medical research will provide a motive for accepting a xenograft. Indeed, respect for individual choice argues that people should be able to offer themselves as experimental subjects, provided that adequate safeguards are in place to ensure that consent is free and properly informed.

7.6 Procedures, which are experimental but offer the chance of genuine treatment for the patients, are termed **therapeutic research.** The important issue is that medical teams should not compromise the care of the individual patient in the interests of scientific research. Rather they must see themselves as using an experimental procedure for which there is evidence that the benefits will outweigh the adverse outcomes. Since clinical trials will take place within the context of a doctor-patient relationship, the doctor is legally obliged to act in the best interests of the patient. Thus, there must be grounds for believing that the treatment will be effective and will offer some benefit to the patient.[1]

7.7 Xenotransplants should therefore be offered to human patients only when results using animal recipients suggest that these operations will have a reasonable chance of success. But it is difficult to say when that stage will have been reached, as a member of a UK team researching xenotransplantation himself has pointed out.[2] There is currently little consensus within the transplantation community, both in the UK and in the US, as to whether the current data using animal recipients justifies progressing

1 Kennedy I and Grubb A (1994) **Medical Law: Text with Materials**, Second edition, pp 1042-3. London: Butterworths.

2 White D (1995) Letter to **Nature**, 378:434.

to clinical trials.[3, 4] Given the difficulty of making this decision, and the importance of not putting patients at unnecessary risk, it would seem advisable that xenotransplantation trials involving human beings should not proceed until there has been an opportunity for consensus amongst the transplantation community to develop, based on discussion of the evidence as published in peer-reviewed scientific and medical journals. Nevertheless, xenotransplant teams have proceeded with trials involving baboon bone marrow in the US.[5] The UK company Imutran Ltd has indicated its intention of starting clinical trials of xenotransplantation using pig organs and tissue in 1996.[6] In contrast, Thomas Starzl, the US transplant surgeon who headed the xenotransplantation of baboon livers into two patients in 1992-3, has argued for a moratorium on further clinical trials of xenotransplantation on the basis that more research is needed before xenotransplantation will be clinically successful.[7]

7.8 The Working Party has recommended the establishment of an Advisory Committee on Xenotransplantation which would regulate xenotransplantation with respect to concerns about the possible transmission of disease-causing organisms (paragraphs 6.38 - 6.41). The proposed Advisory Committee on Xenotransplantation would also have the expertise to assess the success of xenotransplantation using animal models and to advise on when it is scientifically justified to begin clinical trials. **The Working Party recommends that no xenotransplantation trials involving human recipients should proceed until the proposed Advisory Committee on Xenotransplantation is in place and has approved the trials.**

7.9 Local Research Ethics Committees (LRECs) review, and must approve, all proposals for research involving human participants.[8] As such, all proposals for clinical trials of xenotransplantation will be referred to an LREC and will require LREC approval, in addition to the approval of the proposed Advisory Committee on Xenotransplantation.

7.10 This combination of safeguards offered by the proposed Advisory Committee on Xenotransplantation and LRECs would provide a two-fold system for regulating early xenotransplantation trials. This type of system has been successful in regulating gene therapy trials, which require approval from the specially established Gene Therapy Advisory Committee and from LRECs. The Working Party consider that such a system is equally desirable for the regulation of xenotransplantation.

---

3 No cheers for baboon to AIDS patient xenotransplant (1995) **Lancet**, 346:369-70.

4 New ways to avoid organ rejection buoy hopes (1995) **Science, 270**:234-5.

5 AIDS patient given baboon bone marrow (1995) **Nature, 378**:756.

6 Pig-to-human heart transplant slated to begin in 1996 (1995) **Nature Medicine**, 1:987.

7 Starzl T (1995) Comments made at Institute of Medicine conference on Xenograft transplantation: science, ethics and public policy, Washington DC.

8 Department of Health (1991) **Local Research Ethics Committees**, London.

7.11 As set out above, the initial trials to xenotransplant organs will be major and risky procedures. This suggests that it would be justifiable to offer organ xenotransplantation only to patients for whom there is no alternative form of effective treatment. This would apply to many heart patients, whose lives are at risk and for whom the shortage of human organs is acute. The lives of most kidney patients can be maintained, albeit uncomfortably, on dialysis. For some people with renal failure, however, accessing the vascular system becomes extremely difficult and, eventually, dialysis may no longer be possible. The potential, albeit small, risk that xenotransplantation will transmit new infectious diseases to the population at large must also be considered (paragraphs 6.16 - 6.19). It would be hard to justify posing any potential public health risk unless the first xenografts were used to save the lives of people with no alternative possibilities of treatment.

7.12 Another issue is whether it would be unethical to transplant certain types of animal organ or tissues into human beings. One respondent drew a distinction between material "*of a 'mechanical' (for example, heart muscle) rather than 'personal' (for example, neural material) character*".[9] Xenotransplantation of neural tissue has been proposed as a possible treatment for Parkinson's disease. In the US, four Parkinson's disease sufferers have already received xenografts of pig fetal neural cells.[10] It is hoped that the cells of the xenograft will produce the neurotransmitter dopamine that is deficient in Parkinson's sufferers. If successful, this would cause a very specific pharmacological change in the brain. Consequently, the Working Party considers that neural tissue xenografts should be regarded in the same way as any other xenograft intended to restore the body's physical function. Xenotransplantation with the intention of changing aspects of someone's personality is almost certain to remain technically impossible, and would certainly be ethically unacceptable.[11] The unlikely prospect of attempts to alter the germline by xenotransplantation would be equally unacceptable.[12]

7.13 If xenotransplantation of neural tissue were to be successful, it might reduce or eliminate the current use of human fetal neural tissue for transplantation. This material comes from aborted human fetuses and many would see a reduction in its use as desirable. In this respect, some would argue that xenotransplantation would reduce the ethical difficulties associated with neural transplantation. As set out in Chapter 4, however, there is a contrary view that using animals to treat human beings is equally, if not more, unacceptable (paragraph 4.13).

---

9 A point made by Professor John Polkinghorne in his submission to the Working Party.

10 Parkinson's pig cure. **The Times**, 15 December 1995.

11 A view expressed in several submissions to the Working Party including those from the Christian Medical Fellowship, the Church of England and the Methodist Church.

12 A view expressed in submissions from the Joint Ethico-Medical Committee of The Catholic Union of Great Britain and Guild of Catholic Doctors, the Methodist Church, the Royal College of Obstetricians and Gynaecologists.

Consent considerations

7.14 It will be ethically acceptable to offer xenotransplantation to individual patients only when it has been decided, by the procedures set out above, that the results using animal recipients merit starting human trials. At this stage, the question becomes how best to protect early patients' welfare and interests. The principal problems that may arise with the early use of xenografts in human beings include: possible suffering for perhaps limited, if any, therapeutic benefit; the raising of unjustified expectations even when every effort is made to explain honestly the low likelihood of success in early cases; poor quality of life that might follow only a semi-successful use of xenografts; the possibilities of disease transfer across species, which would be an unknowable risk for early patients; and the consequences of the need for health monitoring for those who are recipients. It is likely that the first xenografts will be offered only to those with little chance of surviving without it. But these people, who are facing death, require particular protection from over-optimistic or reckless experiments.

7.15 It is a paramount principle of contemporary medicine that patients should give properly informed consent to any treatment or therapeutic research, and that human volunteers should give properly informed consent to participation in research. People should be in a position to make a decision on the basis of proper information and without pressure, so that participation can truly be said to be voluntary. Where possible, people should make decisions for themselves. Alternative safeguards to protect people who are not considered capable of consenting on their own behalf are considered below (paragraphs 7.22 - 7.26). The Department of Health's 1990 circular, **A guide to consent for examination or treatment**, defines the patient's right to information in the following way:

> "*Patients are entitled to receive sufficient information in a way that they can understand about the proposed treatments, the possible alternatives and any substantial risks, so that they can make a balanced judgement. Patients must be allowed to decide whether they will agree to the treatment, and they may refuse or withdraw consent at any time.*" [13]

7.16 As with any other procedure, it is of the utmost importance that potential patients give free and properly informed consent to participation in the first xenotransplantation trials. The Working Party foresees the following problems with regard to consent to xenotransplantation. First, the risk/benefit ratio of the procedure will be hard to assess in the early stages, because of its novelty. There may be good reason to believe on the basis of experiments using animal recipients that using transgenic animal organs will allow successful xenotransplantation. But

13 NHS Management Executive (1990) **A guide to consent for examination or treatment**. London: Department of Health. p 2.

researchers will only know the risks of the procedure after a considerable number of operations have been carried out in human beings.

7.17 Second, some researchers, keen to discover whether xenografts are a viable alternative to human transplants, might be inclined to overestimate the chance of success. Even with well-established procedures to protect the human subjects of research, innovators may be more dismissive of the risks, and the pains and stresses, of a particular procedure than may be their patients. One North American research programme, for example, discovered that, when men with benign enlargement of the prostate were shown an interactive video, explaining the risks and benefits of surgery, a higher proportion of them chose to postpone surgery (the 'watchful waiting' option) than the surgeons anticipated.[14] If a research team is over-eager to carry out a xenotransplant, its members may naturally find it difficult to present the risk/benefit ratio to the patient in an unbiased way. Subtle changes in the manner of presentation may influence the perception of risk and a patient's decision. For example, one study found that if two treatments are put forward, of equal effectiveness and risk, the alternative presented in terms of the survival rate, rather than the mortality rate, will be consistently preferred by patients and doctors alike, even though both terms describe the same risk, and in this example, the risks of each treatment were the same.[15]

7.18 Thus "*patients must be made aware, whenever possible, of the extent to which they are 'experimental subjects', involved in unpredictable clinical trials of techniques that are largely in the developmental stages.*" [16] To ensure that a patient is given a balanced view, an independent and trained person with appropriate counselling skills, not on the research team wishing to carry out the xenografts, should be given the duty of discussing with the patient the proposed treatment, the possible alternatives and the risks. These discussions should be held as early as is reasonably possible. In order to ensure that consent is properly informed and freely given, **the Working Party recommends that the consent of patients to participation in xenotransplantation trials is sought by appropriately trained professionals who are independent of the xenotransplantation team. The information given to prospective recipients should include an estimation of likely success, attendant risks and subsequent quality of life.**

7.19 As discussed in Chapter 6, it will be extremely important to monitor early xenograft recipients for any evidence that diseases are being transmitted from animals to the early human recipients (paragraphs 6.33 - 6.37). This need to monitor closely the

---

14 Barry M J *et al.* (1988) Watchful waiting versus immediate transurethral resection for symptomatic prostatism: the importance of patients' preferences. **Journal of the American Medical Association,** 259:3010-17.

15 McNeil B J *et al.* (1982) On the elicitation of preferences for alternative therapies. **New England Journal of Medicine,** 306:1259-62.

16 Mepham T and Moore C: submission to the Working Party.

outcomes associated with all early patients brings its own ethical problems, most notably that of how far respect for privacy is consistent with the practice of adequate monitoring. Patients consenting to xenotransplantation should be informed that post-operative monitoring for infectious organisms is an integral part of the procedure, and that their consent to the operation includes consent to this monitoring (paragraph 6.36).

7.20 One piece of information of great importance to patients concerns their expected quality of life. The speed of the body's rejection of xenografts to date has, in most cases, been so fast that quality of life considerations have not arisen (Table 3.1). If xenotransplantation is successful, however, and the patient survives and the xenograft functions properly, quality of life will become important. Teams conducting experimental trials on patients are under a scientific and ethical obligation to research and report the subsequent quality of life of recipients, covering not only post-operative length of life, but also such matters as pain, mobility, emotional adjustment and social functioning. **The Working Party recommends that no protocol to conduct a trial should be accepted unless it contains a commitment to a robust description and assessment of the patient's pre-operative and post-operative quality of life.** Quality of life information should be included in any scientific publication.

7.21 Since xenotransplantation will be an experimental procedure on every occasion on which it is undertaken in the near to medium term, it is essential that those carrying out the procedure report fully on all the important consequences. This will ensure the maximum benefit is obtained from these major and risky procedures. It will improve the information upon which subsequent potential recipients can make a decision. Finally, it will provide more information for public debate on the acceptability of xenotransplantation.

Children

7.22 Special issues arise in the case of children. There is an especially acute shortage of hearts for transplanting into newborn babies with congenital heart defects and of heart-lungs for transplanting into children suffering from cystic fibrosis. It has been suggested that this might justify early xenotransplantation trials involving babies or children: indeed, in 1984 in the US, a baboon heart was transplanted into Baby Fae.[17] She survived 20 days.

17 Baily L L *et al.* (1985) Baboon-to-human cardiac xenotransplantation in a neonate. **Journal of the American Medical Association,** 254:3321.

7.23 As discussed above, therapeutic research must offer some benefit to the patient (paragraph 7.6). Since, by its nature, however, therapeutic research involves greater uncertainties than treatment, greater caution must be exercised. The British Paediatric Association and the Medical Research Council have advised that therapeutic research should not involve children if it could equally well be performed with adults.[18, 19] In the case of early xenotransplantation trials, the main problem is likely to be overcoming organ rejection, which will be a problem in both adults and children. Thus, it would be difficult to justify the involvement of children in major and risky trials as recipients of heart xenografts, for example, before some of the uncertainties have been eliminated in trials involving adults. **The Working Party recommends that the first xenotransplantation trials involve adults rather than children.**

7.24 The special protection afforded children needs to be balanced with the importance of not withholding potentially beneficial treatment, even if that benefit is offered in the context of therapeutic research. If the first adult trials are successful, and there is greater certainty about the benefits, there would be stronger arguments for offering xenotransplantation to children. The question of consent then becomes important. Children between 16 and 18 may be considered capable of consenting on their own behalf to participate in therapeutic research, although a higher level of maturity would probably be required than that needed for consent to medical treatment. Given the complexity of the ethics and law in this area, a cautious approach would be to obtain the consent of the person with parental responsibility before a child under 18 participates in a major procedure like xenotransplantation.[20, 21] The agreement of any child to participation in therapeutic research such as xenotransplantation should always be obtained.

Adults who cannot consent on their own behalf

7.25 Similar issues arise for adults who are considered incapable of consenting to participation in therapeutic research because they are mentally incapacitated. The law would appear to be that incapacitated adults may be involved in therapeutic research if this is in their best interests.[22] In its study of the law relating to mental incapacity, the Law Commission recommended that therapeutic research should be

---

18 British Paediatric Association (1992) **Guidelines for the Ethical Conduct of Medical Research Involving Children.**

19 Medical Research Council (1991) **MRC Ethics Series: The Ethical Conduct of Research on Children.** London.

20 Kennedy I and Grubb A (1994) **Medical Law: Text with Materials** Second edition. London: Butterworths, p 1043.

21 Department of Health (1991) **Local research ethics committees,** London. p 16.

22 Kennedy I and Grubb A (1994) **Medical Law: Text with Materials** Second edition. London: Butterworths, pp 1052-4.

lawful *"if it is in all the circumstances reasonable"*.[23] It would be difficult to justify, by this standard, the involvement of incapacitated adults in the first xenotransplantation trials before some of the major uncertainties have been eliminated in trials involving adults who are capable of weighing the benefits and risks on their own behalf. **The Working Party recommends that the first xenotransplantation trials should not involve adults incapable of consenting to participation on their own behalf.**

7.26 The Medical Research Council has recommended that the participation of incapacitated adults in therapeutic research may be justified if, in addition to evidence that the procedure will benefit the individual, it relates to their incapacitating condition and the relevant knowledge could not be gained by research in adults able to consent.[24] One situation in which this might justify xenotransplantation trials involving the mentally incapacitated is the proposed transplantation of pig fetal neural tissue to treat people suffering from Huntington's disease, a neurodegenerative disorder which affects mental capacity. Such trials should only take place, however, if there is evidence to support progressing from animal research to human trials and to indicate that the procedure will benefit the individuals involved.

Conscientious objections

7.27 One of the starting points for this report was that public policy must reflect the ethical pluralism that characterises this and many other societies (paragraph 1.29). In Chapter 4, the Working Party concluded that xenotransplantation using organs and tissue from transgenic pigs would be ethically acceptable (paragraphs 4.42 and 4.49). Some people, however, will conscientiously hold the opinion that xenotransplantation is wrong in principle. Some of these people will themselves turn out to be eligible for xenotransplantation should the technology turn out to be feasible. By the principle of consent, they would be quite entitled to refuse a xenograft for this or any other reason such as religious, cultural or ethical grounds or, indeed, because they do not think the benefits of xenotransplantation outweigh the risks.

7.28 What are the implications for people who refuse xenografts? This may become an important issue if xenotransplantation develops into a successful procedure. Xenotransplantation might then offer a cheaper form of treatment than, say, dialysis for patients with kidney failure. There might, then, be pressure on individuals to accept xenografts. Certainly, patients must always be told the sources of the organ

---

23 Law Commission Report No 231 (1995) **Mental Incapacity** London: HMSO. See in particular pp 49-51.

24 Medical Research Council (1991) **MRC Ethics Series: The Ethical Conduct of Research on the Mentally Incapacitated.** London.

or tissue they might receive: withholding such information would amount to deception. Another issue is how refusal of a xenograft might affect an individual's consideration for human organ transplantation.

7.29 Consider the situation in which refusing a xenograft reduced a person's priority for receiving a human organ, presumably on the grounds that they had been offered, and refused, an appropriate form of treatment. In this case, consent to xenotransplantation certainly would not be freely given. Rather, an element of coercion would be involved. The principle of respect for conscientious objection would be compromised if people who objected had to accept greater harm than others.

7.30 Should people who refuse xenografts be given some priority in access to human organs, in order not to jeopardise their freedom of conscience? In some cases, such as the refusal of blood transfusion by a Jehovah's Witness, refusal of treatment will result in a greater risk to the patient and so there can be little doubt of the patient's sincerity. But objection to xenotransplantation might be seen as self-interested if, by refusing a xenograft, that person were given priority for a human organ transplant. **The Working Party recommends that at any stage in the development of xenotransplantation, patients who, for whatever reasons, refuse xenografts should remain entitled to consideration for human organs on the same basis as before their refusal.**

7.31 A question then arises about what should happen to the status of a person who has accepted a xenograft, but for whom a human transplant at some later date might offer better prospects. In the early stages of development, xenografts are unlikely to be as successful as human transplants, and it is possible that they will only work for a fairly short period of time. At least initially, xenotransplantation might be used as a bridging procedure to keep a patient alive until a human organ became available.[25] This suggests that, in principle, accepting a xenograft should not affect the recipient's entitlement should a suitable human organ become available. It is true that, in practice, receiving a xenograft might affect the suitability of the person for a subsequent human organ transplantation, in terms of their physical fitness, for example. This does not, however, seem unfair. Other factors, such as the degree of tissue matching, being equal, human organs are made available on the basis of clinical need. All patients would have the opportunity to accept or to refuse a xenograft, fully informed of the consequences of so doing. **The Working Party recommends that xenograft recipients should remain entitled to consideration for human organ transplantation on the same basis of clinical need as before xenotransplantation.** The Working Party recognises that an implication of this position is that the demand for human organs may not decline, and may even

25 Steele D and Auchincloss H (1995) The application of xenotransplantation in humans - reasons to delay. **Institute of Laboratory Animal Resources Journal**, 37:13-5.

increase, in the early years of xenotransplantation, since xenograft recipients may remain on the waiting list for human organs whereas without a xenograft they might not have survived.

Health care workers

7.32 It is not only patients who may have conscientious objections to involvement with xenografts. The right of conscientious objection should also be extended to health care personnel. In this case, the right cannot be understood to be absolute. Rather, it must be seen as a consideration which should always be taken seriously by other medical and managerial personnel in individual cases. Problems are unlikely to arise in the early stages of xenografts, since they will be carried out in special centres, staffed, presumably, by people who do not object to xenotransplantation. But in later stages it may be considered reasonable, perhaps, for a nurse to refuse to participate in the actual xenograft, but not, say, to refuse to take food to a recipient of a xenograft. As set out in Chapter 6, there is a case for monitoring health care workers involved in xenotransplantation for the possible transmission of animal diseases (paragraph 6.34). This requirement should be made clear to all involved.

7.33 The question also arises of what responsibilities medical personnel would have were it to become clear that involvement with xenografts was dangerous for them, perhaps because of the risk of infection. In entering the profession, health care workers assume a duty to accept certain reasonable risks, especially when efficient protective measures are available. Thus, health care workers are expected to care for people infected with the HIV virus, and, similarly, they might be expected to care for people suffering from diseases transmitted via xenotransplantation. In extreme cases, however, it cannot be demanded of any member of staff that they place themselves at severe risk. In the unlikely event that xenotransplantation leads to the emergence of a highly infectious disease, the only solution would be to call for volunteers.

Conclusion

7.34 This chapter has set out the following ethical issues that need to be taken into account in the regulation of xenotransplantation involving human recipients:

- the timing of the first trials
- consent considerations
- conscientious objection

These concerns will best be taken account of if clinical trials of xenotransplantation are restricted initially to a small number of approved centres. The decision to proceed with clinical trials involving human beings will also require an assessment of whether concerns about infectious organisms have been addressed adequately (paragraph 6.41). This is an important concern both for individual patients, and for the wider population. The Working Party considers that it would not be ethical to undertake clinical trials of xenotransplantation until a regulatory structure is in place that can take account of all these concerns. This reinforces the argument for an Advisory Committee on Xenotransplantation.

Chapter 8

Effects on the health care system

Implications for the National Health Service

8.1 The purpose of the National Health Service (NHS) is to improve health, as measured in terms of both the quality and the length of life. If the development of xenotransplantation overcomes the scientific hurdles described in Chapter 3, satisfies the ethical considerations set out in Chapters 4 to 7 and offers real benefits to individuals at an acceptable level of risk to the population as a whole, then the NHS is likely pursue its introduction. If xenografting becomes a viable clinical treatment, it will join a long list of innovations. Adapting to technological change has been an abiding theme for the NHS since its inception in 1948.

8.2 The NHS was established just as sulphonamides and antibiotics were beginning to offer medicine an apparent mastery over infectious diseases. Since then, a succession of changes in diagnosis and treatment has transformed medical practice. No branch of health care has remained unchanged: psychotropic pharmaceutical treatments have radically altered psychiatry since the 1950s; dialysis programmes have meant the introduction of treatments for people with previously untreatable kidney failure; and hip and knee replacements, along with organ transplantation programmes themselves, offer therapeutic alternatives to processes of degeneration, decay and death that to previous generations were inevitable. Currently, the NHS is grappling with the implications of the introduction of beta-interferon, an expensive drug that may alleviate the effects of multiple sclerosis in a proportion of sufferers.[1, 2]

8.3 The NHS has had to meet considerable challenges in introducing and disseminating major programmes of technological change. This has included coping with the cost and organisational impact of changed clinical practice. New requirements have been established for training, as well as for expenditure on buildings and equipment. The effects of this are demonstrable: the fever hospitals and tuberculosis wards characteristic of the service in the late 1940s have given way to intensive care suites and units devoted to day cases and minimally invasive surgery in the 1990s.

---

1 Walley, Barton S (1995) A purchaser perspective of managing new drugs: interferon beta as a case study **British Medical Journal**, 311:796-9.

2 Multiple sclerosis drug prompts rationing fears (1995) **British Medical Journal,** 311:969.

8.4 Such change has generally happened incrementally and without a well-rounded assessment of the benefits and costs of particular innovations, although the system of limiting major innovations like dialysis and organ transplantation to regional and/or national centres has permitted a measured introduction of certain techniques. Given the nature of innovation in treatments, an element of ad hoc incrementalism is all but inevitable. The full benefits of innovations can often be assessed only when they have been in place for some time: no one, looking at the first results from the early experiments in heart transplantation in the 1960s could have foreseen either their benefits to individual transplant recipients or their cost to the public purse.

8.5 The allocation of resources within the NHS is currently a matter of intense debate and widespread concern.[3,4] Xenotransplantation, like any expensive new technology, will intensify this wider problem. In this context, it is important to consider the potential impact of xenotransplantation on the NHS, should it move beyond the experimental stage to the point where it is a routine surgical procedure. At present, it is not possible to answer this question in any detail. But in this chapter some of the key issues are set out.

The cost of xenotransplantation compared with human organ transplantation

8.6 As noted in the opening chapter, the cost of present transplantation procedures is not that high, when compared with other types of treatment (paragraph 1.6). How will the costs of xenotransplantation compare with these existing costs? The present cost of transplantation is due, largely, to the cost of transplant operations and the cost of drugs for preventing the rejection of transplanted organs. In addition, there are costs that arise from the system used to obtain organs from human donors. These include the costs associated with contributing to the maintenance of intensive care units and the costs of coordinating the supply of organs.

8.7 Xenotransplantation will not lead to a reduction in many of these costs. The cost of the operation will be about the same, except that the organ or tissue will have to be bought. Human organs are freely donated, although there are costs of caring for donors, and the collection, maintenance and coordination of organs prior to transplantation. These costs are unlikely to decrease in the near future since the use of human organs is likely to be the preferred procedure. So it will still be necessary to contribute to the upkeep of intensive care units and to keep coordination arrangements in place. In contrast to human organs, xenografted organs would not be free at source. The cost of an organ from a transgenic pig is likely to be high,

3 Klein R (1995) Priorities and rationing; pragmatism or principles? **British Medical Journal**, 311:761-2.

4 Maxwell R ed. (1995) Rationing Health Care. **British Medical Bulletin**, 55:761-962.

reflecting the cost of the innovation required to produce it, as well as the cost of breeding and rearing animals in the required conditions. If, however, xenotransplantation became a successful procedure and large numbers of organs were supplied, the individual cost of each organ supplied should fall. The cost of such organs, however, would be a new charge on the NHS, as would the costs of monitoring xenograft recipients for evidence of infection with disease-causing organisms (paragraphs 6.33 - 6.37).

8.8 It is likely that, at least initially, xenotransplanted organs will require levels of immunosuppression at least equal to that necessary for human organs. It has been argued, however, that the development of transgenic animals will result in animal organs and tissue that require lower levels of immunosuppression than are required for human organs and tissue.[5] If so, this would reduce the costs of immunosuppressive drugs for xenotransplant recipients.

The scope of xenotransplantation

8.9 If xenotransplantation becomes a successful clinical procedure, then transplantation programmes are likely to expand greatly, since they will no longer be constrained by the shortage of human organs. More people will receive transplants. These will include patients who are currently eligible for transplantation but who are not fortunate enough to be recipients of a human organ. Thus, for kidney transplants, basing an estimate on the most recent information about the numbers of transplants performed and the numbers of people waiting for treatment, the cost might increase to about four times the cost of the present programme.[6] Although this would represent a significant change in the size of the transplant programme itself, this increase in costs could be relatively easily absorbed within the total budget of the NHS.

8.10 Because of the human organ shortage, some people are currently not considered for transplantation. At the moment, transplantation is offered only to those who are both sufficiently seriously ill to need an organ and for whom there is a reasonably good chance of transplantation being successful. Among those excluded at present are people whose prognosis is not too poor and who are being treated with drugs, and those over a certain age for whom the clinical prognosis is not as good as for younger patients. Xenotransplantation, might allow transplants to be offered to a much larger number of people. For example, heart transplants could be offered to elderly patients with cardiac failure caused by coronary artery disease, whereas at

5 Cozzi E and White D J G (1995) The generation of transgenic pigs as potential organ donors for humans. **Nature Medicine,** 1:964-6.

6 1,744 transplants were performed in 1994, and nearly three times that number, 4,970 people, remained on the waiting list (paragraph 1.7).

present only younger people are considered as having a high priority for human organs. While the health benefits of this could be considerable, the cost of transplantation programmes overall would be likely to increase. It is difficult to predict how far xenotransplantation might become the preferred mode of treatment for people who are not currently considered for human organ transplantation: potentially, this could lead to a large increase in transplantation activity.

8.11 Finally, transplantation procedures might be extended to a larger number of organs and tissues in the body, since the ready supply of organs and tissue will make it easier to develop and implement new procedures. There is much interest, for example, in the use of pig fetal neural tissue transplants for treating neurodegenerative diseases (paragraph 3.35). Such an expansion in transplantation activity would also increase the costs of the service.

8.12 The effects of xenotransplantation outside the transplantation service also need to be considered. For example, an increase in kidney transplantation would reduce the numbers of people on long-term dialysis, which is an expensive treatment (paragraph 1.6). The costs of drugs for the treatment of disease and the cost of hospital stays for those with failing organs might also be expected to decrease if organ and tissue replacement by xenotransplantation were to increase.

Arrangements for introducing xenotransplantation into the NHS

8.13 Based on the discussion above, it is likely that the major cost implications of xenotransplantation would arise from the larger number of transplants that will be possible if the shortage of organs and tissue is overcome. These costs are difficult to estimate but they could be considerable. The main constraint on transplant programmes at the moment is not cost but the shortage of human organs and tissue. Should xenotransplantation develop into successful procedure and reduce this shortage, decisions about its provision will have to be made within the context of the wider debate about how resources are allocated within the NHS. As with other treatments, such as assisted reproduction and beta-interferon, there will be difficult choices to be made about priorities and rationing.[7, 8] The Methodist Church wrote in their submission: "*The cost effectiveness of major work on transplants using genetically engineered animal sources must be judged against the health gain which could be achieved by a similar investment in preventive medicine, public health programmes and amelioration of poor social conditions.*"

7 Multiple sclerosis drug prompts rationing fears (1995) **British Medical Journal**, 311:969.

8 Survey shows widespread rationing in NHS (1995) **British Medical Journal**, 311:1453-4.

8.14 The development of xenotransplantation into a successful clinical procedure, however, is some way in the future. This will allow the NHS to control its introduction and to assess it carefully. Research teams currently developing xenotransplantation should keep accurate and accountable records of the costs of the procedures. In this way, policy makers will be in a better position to assess the cost implications. Should xenotransplantation cease to be experimental and become feasible as a clinical treatment, it should be restricted to designated centres for the foreseeable future. This would ensure adequate control of costs and monitoring of cost-effectiveness.

8.15 One model for the provision of specialist services in the NHS is the Supra Regional Services Advisory Group. This Advisory Group is responsible for 10 designated specialist services including the Heart, Heart-Lung and Lung Transplant Service and the Liver Transplant Service. The Advisory Group was established as a result of the 1991 NHS reforms with the following terms of reference:

> *"To advise the Secretary of State, through Regional Chairmen of Health Authorities, on the identification of services to be funded supra regionally and on the appropriate level of provision."* [9]

Any such service is expected to meet the following criteria. It must:

- *"already be an established clinical (not diagnostic) service and offer the treatment of choice;*
- *cover a condition which is sufficiently rare that the service should only be provided by any single unit for a population significantly larger than 5 million;*
- *relate to a clearly defined group of patients with a condition whose rarity is such that the national caseload would not exceed 1,000 and would normally be about 400 a year;*
- *be capable of being provided in a small number of centres which between them can meet the national caseload and that the profession would accept that the service should only be provided in a restricted number of centres;*
- *be able to justify its costs when set against alternative uses for NHS funds; and*
- *cost such an amount that it would constitute a significant burden for providers and purchasers."* [10]

---

9 Supra Regional Services Advisory Group annual report (1994-5) p 6.

10 Supra Regional Services Advisory Group annual report (1994-5) p 7.

8.16 From 1 April 1996, the Supra Regional Services Advisory Group will have additional responsibilities including "*funding the service costs of new developments, in those services for which it is the purchaser, to enable full evaluation to take place*". This would allow the involvement of the Supra Regional Services Advisory Group in the provision of services, such as xenotransplantation, before they are established clinical services.[11]

8.17 A mechanism such as the Supra Regional Services Advisory Group would allow the introduction and provision of xenotransplantation which, at the outset, will be a rare and expensive treatment, in a controlled way. **The Working Party recommends that, if xenotransplantation becomes a treatment of choice, the introduction of the treatment into the NHS should be overseen by the Supra Regional Services Advisory Group.** The Supra Regional Services Advisory Group would be concerned with administration and financing and thus its role would be distinct from that of the proposed Advisory Committee on Xenotransplantation responsible for establishing good practice in xenotransplantation (paragraph 6.41).

11 Supra Regional Services Advisory Group annual report (1994-5) p 3. The Group's name will change to National Specialist Commissioning Advisory Group to reflect these additional responsibilities.

Chapter 9

Personal and social effects of xenotransplantation

9.1 A health care system is part of a wider social order. Developments in health care cannot, therefore, be separated from their social context and the broader effects they may have. It is difficult to predict how social attitudes and institutions will respond to xenotransplantation, should it become introduced as a clinical treatment. It is important to consider what these responses might be, however, even if there is, inevitably, an element of speculation involved. In this chapter, therefore, the broader social implications of xenotransplantation are considered.

Attitudes towards xenotransplantation

9.2 One view of xenotransplantation is that it represents yet another attempt by human beings to deny their own mortality. Susan Roberts wrote in her submission: "*For whilst the improvement in medical techniques is an admirable challenge to face, we do appear to be driven by an overriding desire to fight death at all costs. Perhaps if we could come to terms with the forces of nature at work within our own lives, it would enable us to reach a position of equanimity with the rest of the planet.*" This view reflects a more general ambivalence about 'high-tech' medicine that is sometimes thought not only to yield little benefit in terms of increased quality of life but also to undermine human dignity in death.[1] Survey respondents, for example, often express a preference for treatments that reduce pain or disability over those that add a little to the length of life. These reservations extend to human organ transplantation. There is also concern about the morality of practices associated with obtaining human organs for transplantation (paragraphs 2.6 - 2.10). Underlying these attitudes is a sense of the inherent limitations of modern medicine, and a recognition that death can be staved off a little but never defeated. In this context, xenotransplantation can be regarded as part of the quest to prolong life, in pursuit of which goal, human beings are prepared to abuse their relationship with other animals.

9.3 Transplantation does not have to be regarded, however, as a form of heroic intervention that strives to extend life at any cost, with little regard to the best interests of the patient. As discussed in Chapter 1, transplantation is increasingly a routine, and not especially expensive, form of treatment that offers significant

1 Calman M and Williams S (1992) Images of scientific medicine. **Sociology of Health and Illness, 14:233-54.**

improvements in length and quality of life and, were it not for the organ shortage, could do so for a large number of people. In this context, xenotransplantation if clinically effective, might offer a way of alleviating the organ shortage that would reduce the need for controversial measures to increase the supply of human organs. The use of animals, while undesirable, might be seen as raising ethical difficulties less severe than those that arise in solving the organ shortage by other means (Chapter 2). In a study of young people's attitudes to xenografts in the UK, while concerns were expressed about this use of animals, 55 per cent considered that research to develop pig organs for transplantation should continue (45 per cent opposed it).[2] Many of the those who wrote to the Working Party expressed profound sympathy for the plight of people in need of treatment and the hope that xenotransplantation might offer a solution. These views were combined with a recognition of the need for safeguards to ensure the protection of both human beings and animals (paragraph 1.32).

9.4 The concerns expressed about medical developments in general, and about transplantation and xenotransplantation in particular, highlight the importance of transparency and openness in the activities of researchers and policy-makers involved in xenotransplantation, and of full debate across society about its acceptability. The National Spiritual Assembly of the Bahá'ís of the UK stressed the importance of ongoing consultation and the "*seeking of the views of the wider community.*" If these measures are fulfilled, attitudes to xenotransplantation will reflect informed and considered opinion. This should also reduce any danger that xenograft recipients would be stigmatised in any way.

Effects of xenotransplantation for individual recipients

9.5 An important question is how xenotransplantation might affect individual recipients. A person's self-image is clearly related to their perception of the body. When assessing the impact of xenotransplantation, it will be necessary to consider how a person's perception of their body, and of their identity or self-image, is affected. A person's sense of identity also depends on a history of involvement with other persons, as well as with other elements, both animate and inanimate, of the environment. Thus, the impact of xenotransplantation will depend to an extent on the responses of health care workers, carers, family members and others close to xenograft recipients. Any assessment of xenotransplantation should take into account its potential impact on these relationships.

2 This was part of a project funded under the BIOTECH programmes entitled **Cultural and Social Objections to Biotechnology: analysis of the arguments with special reference to the views of young people.** Dr Mairi Levitt described the project in her submission to the Working Party: 238 students, aged 11-18 years, from three different schools were given background material about xeno- transplantation and then answered a questionnaire.

9.6 In trying to assess how people might adapt to xenotransplantation, it is helpful to draw on research that has examined the personal impact of human organ transplantation.[3] This research indicates that how well, or badly, someone adapts to transplantation can have a significant impact on physical recovery and on health. In particular, there may be a direct effect on the level of compliance with the demanding regime of immuno-suppressive drugs and other follow-up procedures needed by transplant recipients.

9.7 The stresses of human organ transplantation fall into two classes: those experienced before transplantation, and those occurring afterwards.[4] The stresses before transplantation include dealing with the effects of a severe illness, and coping with the long wait for a transplant and the uncertainty of a suitable organ or tissue becoming available whilst being close to death.[5] If xenotransplantation succeeds in alleviating the shortage of organs for transplantation, making transplantation available more quickly and to more people, these stresses might be significantly reduced.

9.8 Stresses occurring as a consequence of transplantation include the general stresses of hospitalisation and surgery. More specific stresses include coping with the fear of rejection of the transplant or with infection; with the intrusive nature of immunosuppression and follow-up treatment; and with a change in image of the body.[6] Different levels of significance are attached to different transplants: tissue transplantation, for example is seen as much less significant than organ transplantation. Heart transplantation is seen as most significant, since so much symbolic importance is attached to that organ: "*It is the seat of emotions (especially love) courage, enthusiasm and innermost thoughts.*" [7] Transplant recipients report being affected by thoughts of organ donors and their families. For some, it is disturbing that they have inside them an organ from someone who has died.[8]

9.9 There is evidence that transplantation is particularly stressful for children and adolescents.[9] Young children may not understand why they are ill, and may perceive it as punishment. Self-image and the peer group are particularly important for adolescents, and this may lead to problems with adjusting to receiving a transplant, coping with scars and the physical side-effects of immunosuppressive drugs. Adolescents' increased desire for independence may lead to resentment of the

---

3 Craven J and Rodin G M (1992) **Psychiatric Aspects of Organ Transplantation.** New York: Oxford Medical Publications.

4 Craven and Rodin (1992) **Psychiatric Aspects of Organ Transplantation,** pp 90-7.

5 British Heart Foundation (1995) **Cardiac Transplantation.**

6 Craven and Rodin (1992) **Psychiatric Aspects of Organ Transplantation,** pp 95-7.

7 Submission to the Working Party from the Working Group on Genetic Engineering in Non-human Life Forms of the Society, Religion & Technology Project of the Church of Scotland.

8 Craven and Rodin (1992) **Psychiatric Aspects of Organ Transplantation,** pp 169-71.

9 Craven and Rodin (1992) **Psychiatric Aspects of Organ Transplantation,** pp 33-49.

restrictions associated with immunosuppressive drug regimes and problems with compliance.

9.10 How might the stresses of xenotransplantation compare with those of human organ transplantation? For early recipients, at least, fear of transplant rejection is likely to be very real. Follow-up will also be very demanding, since it will involve procedures to monitor possible transmission of animal diseases (paragraphs 6.33 - 6.37). Compliance, or otherwise, with such monitoring will have implications not just for the health of the individual recipients, but possibly for the wider community.

9.11 It is difficult to predict how people's views of their bodies and of their identities, might be affected by xenotransplantation. On the one hand, the use of animal organs might eliminate any disturbing implications associated with receiving a human organ. On the other hand, receiving an animal transplant might cause different stresses. The response is likely to reflect notions of what it is to be a person, to be human and to be an animal. These notions are not uniform for this or any other society, but vary according to social and cultural background. A small UK survey has shown that 40 per cent of potential recipients would have no objection to receiving a pig kidney. A US survey of transplant recipients found that they were more likely to say they would accept a xenograft if they needed another transplant and no human organ was available.[10] An Australian survey of acute care nurses found that two-thirds said they would not accept transplantation of an organ from a pig.[11]

9.12 One cause of unease is the breaching of normally inviolate boundaries.[12, 13] This is seen in human organ transplantation. The recipient of a transplanted organ may feel that the boundary between self and non-self has been breached. As described above, receiving an organ from a dead person may also disturb the recipient. With xenotransplantation, an additional boundary, that between human and animal, may become blurred. Whether, or in what ways, this is perceived as a problem will depend on how the human being-animal boundary is defined and the significance that is attached to it. If the essence of humanity is seen as a capacity to transcend the level of organic existence, then a person's sense of identity should not, in theory, be threatened by a transfer of organs across species boundaries. The idea of xenotransplantation may become troublesome if there is not thought to be a strict division between humanity and bodily existence. In this case, to receive an organ

---

10 The UK study was carried out at Guy's and St Thomas's Medical and Dental School, London and presented at the British Renal Symposium, Harrogate in 1994. The US study was carried out by the National Kidney Foundation (NKF Survey reveals positive feelings on animal-to-human transplants (1995) **Dialysis and Transplantation,** December 1995, p 677). These surveys were described in the submission from the UK National Kidney Federation.

11 Mohacsi P *et al.* (1995) Letter to **Nature**, 378:434.

12 This section draws on the submissions from Marilyn Strathern and Tania Woods.

13 Fox R (1995) Presentation at an Institute of Medicine conference on Xenograft transplantation: science, ethics and public policy, Washington DC.

from another animal might be seen as a mixing of one's human essence with that of the animal, and therefore as a dilution of one's humanity. Xenotransplantation will be troublesome for a different reason if it is felt that some or all of those characteristics by which human beings are recognised as persons are also shared by animals (paragraph 4.13). To receive organs or tissue obtained by killing a healthy animal might then be seen as objectionable.

9.13 It is sometimes argued that if receiving an animal transplant was particularly disturbing to pig heart valve recipients this would have emerged as a problem by now. As mentioned above, however, the significance of a transplant varies, depending on the particular organ or tissue (paragraph 9.8). Pig heart valves are small pieces of tissue that have been treated to make them non-viable. The possibility that someone might react much more strongly to transplantation of a vital organ from an animal cannot be dismissed.

9.14 The submissions received by the Working Party contained a range of reactions to the idea of xenotransplantation. Sheila Silcock asked "*Might there be such a thing as emotional rejection? Suppose a patient suddenly had a revulsion about having received an animal organ. Counselling prior to organ transplant is essential and would presumably be even more vital before a xenotransplant.*" Audrey McLaughlan reported that "*patients in the Renal Unit mentioned that they had qualms about having animal organs within their bodies.*" Students from Dalriada School in Northern Ireland had a variety of opinions. Some said: "*I would be prepared to accept an organ from a pig.*" and "*using a pig organ in your body is better than dying.*" Others said: "*we have been made superior to animals and it would be degrading to be made of part pig, part human*" and "*the concept of an organ being part of me seems quite distasteful*". How xenotransplantation might be regarded by people who view the pig as ritually unclean was discussed in Chapter 4 (paragraph 4.24).

9.15 Predicting how people might feel if xenotransplantation were performed on them or on someone close to them, is very difficult. Virtually nothing is known about the effects of xenotransplantation upon perceptions of identity, whether for xenograft recipients or amongst those who care for them or interact with them in other ways. This highlights the need for more research into these issues. **The Working Party recommends that counselling of xenograft recipients should include discussion of the possible personal impact of xenotransplantation. The Working Party further recommends that research should be initiated to study the personal impact of xenotransplantation on potential and early recipients.**

The implications of xenotransplantation for attitudes to human organ donation

9.16 An important concern raised by xenotransplantation is the possible effect upon willingness to donate human organs. Relatives and friends will often find solace in the knowledge that the death of a loved one has not been entirely futile but has given the gift of life to another. The organisation called BODY has been established to bring together relatives of donors. They provide examples of families who say that it has been a great comfort to them to know that the organs of a loved one have given life to someone else.[14] In one case, parents who agreed to the transplantation of their dead son's kidney value an anonymous letter from the recipient's mother as among their most treasured possessions. The gratitude of recipients is also striking. One liver transplant patient has said that not a day goes by without her thinking of the person whose liver she received.[15] Thus, the present system of human donation creates a delicate web of relationships among members of society that reflects a commitment to social solidarity and mutual concern.

9.17 The willingness of human beings to donate their organs, however, is hard to sustain (paragraphs 2.7 - 2.8). Quite a small amount of adverse publicity will have large effects on rates of organ donation. Conversely, it is an uphill struggle to increase the number of people registered as organ donors, even despite initiatives such as the NHS Organ Donor Register.[16] It appears that the ethical concerns and anxieties people have about organ donation are only partly overcome by the sense that organ donation is the ultimate gift in that it allows someone else to live.

9.18 In this context, there is a danger that xenotransplantation could jeopardise the willingness with which human organs are donated. This may be for two reasons. Firstly, early publicity about successful xenografts could lead potential donors or relatives to think that it was no longer worthwhile to register for organ donation; people might assume that the use of animal organs had eliminated the need for human organs. Secondly, unease at xenotransplantation might increase the general concerns about organ transplantation and lead to a fall in the donation of human organs.

9.19 It is highly unlikely, however, that xenotransplantation will eliminate the need for human organs. In the near future, at least, xenografts are unlikely to be as successful as human organ transplants. The most likely outcome is that xenotransplantation will ultimately become part of a range of strategies that could be used in the

14 The British Organ Donor Society (BODY) (1991) **The Gift of Life: An introduction to organ and tissue transplantation.**

15 Brooks G (1995) Comments at an Institute of Medicine conference on Xenograft transplantation: science, ethics and public policy, Washington DC.

16 For information about the NHS Organ Donor Register, freephone 0800 555777.

treatment of organ failure, alongside human organ transplantation, and the use of artificial or bioengineered substitutes. It is very important, therefore, to indicate to potential and actual donors that their gift is no less precious because a development involving animals has now become part of the repertoire of treatment. A particular concern is that xenografts are unlikely to be uniformly successful across different organs and tissue. For example, the use of animal organs for liver transplants presents more difficulties than the use of animal organs for heart transplants because of the liver's complicated biochemistry (paragraph 3.6). Thus, it will remain essential to maintain levels of human organ donation.

9.20 There is a great responsibility, therefore, on xenotransplant teams, on the media and on those responsible for influencing public opinion to ensure that the reporting of developments in xenografts is as accurate, balanced and unsensational as possible. The temptation must be resisted to report early animal or clinical trials as scientific breakthroughs that presage a speedy solution to the problems created by the shortage of human organs. It should be clear from this report that, for the foreseeable future, xenotransplantation will not solve the shortage of organs for transplantation and that there will still be a pressing need for the donation of human organs.

Conclusions and recommendations

Chapter 10

Conclusions and recommendations

10.1 There is considerable interest in the transplantation of animal organs or tissue as a means of reducing the shortage of human organs and tissue for transplantation. Transplantation is an important and successful procedure in modern health care. It provides significant benefits to patients, both extending life expectancy and improving quality of life (Chapter 1). Debate continues about how to reduce the gap between the demand for transplantation and the shortage of human organs and tissue (Chapter 2). The benefits of preventive measures to improve health and prevent the diseases requiring treatment by transplantation are likely to be long-term ones (paragraphs 2.2 - 2.3). Some of the suggested measures for increasing the supply of human organs, such as changing the consent requirements, are not without ethical and practical difficulties (paragraphs 2.4 - 2.10). Even radically innovative measures to increase rates of human organ donation are likely to be insufficient to bridge the gap between supply and demand. The gap is, if anything, likely to widen, not least because improvements in surgical and medical techniques will permit a larger range of patients to be treated by transplantation.

10.2 Thus, there is interest in alternative ways of meeting the organ shortage. Mechanical devices, notably battery-powered hearts, have made great advances in recent years, and may be expected to develop further (paragraphs 2.11 - 2.21). They are prone to problems, however, associated with increased risks of infection and of blood clotting. Mechanical devices are also unlikely to be able to take the place of some human organs, such as the liver, which has sophisticated biochemical functions. Tissue engineering techniques, in which living cells are used to produce replacement organs and tissue, are promising, but still in the early stages of development (paragraphs 2.22 - 2.31). Skin can now be replaced by tissue engineering, but the development of bioengineered heart valves, much less functioning organs, is a more distant prospect.

10.3 Xenotransplantation of animal organs and tissues is an alternative option for reducing the shortage of human organs and tissue for transplantation. The strong immune response to animal organs or tissue, however, means that transplant rejection is a major problem and, to date, xenotransplantation involving human recipients has not been successful (Table 3.1). An exception is the routine transplantation of pig heart valves. These can be treated so they do not cause such a strong immune response. Two main strategies have been used to try and prevent xenograft rejection. In the US, attempts have been made to use organs and tissue from primates, such as baboons, for xenotransplantation. Since, biologically speaking, primates are closely related to human beings, the immune response to a primate xenograft is not that much stronger than the response to a poorly matched human transplant. In December 1995, an AIDS sufferer from the US received a transplant of baboon bone marrow in the hope that this would restore the function of his bone marrow (paragraphs 3.18 - 3.21).

10.4 Ethical concerns about the use of primates for xenotransplantation have led to attempts to develop non-primates as sources of organs and tissue. Attention has focused in particular on pigs, since their organs are comparable in size to human ones, and they breed rapidly and could thus be used to supply transplant material on a large scale. Since pigs are less closely related to human beings than primates, the immune response to pig xenografts is rapid and severe. Attempts are being made to modify pigs genetically so that their organs do not cause such a strong immune response when transplanted into human beings (paragraphs 3.24 - 3.32). Hearts from these transgenic pigs last longer than unmodified organs when they are transplanted into monkeys. The UK company Imutran Ltd has announced its intention to start transplanting hearts from transgenic pigs into human recipients in 1996. In the US, Parkinson's sufferers have undergone xenotransplantation of fetal neural tissue from unmodified pigs in an attempt to treat their condition (paragraph 3.35).

Ethical concerns

10.5 Given the recent developments in overcoming the problems associated with xenotransplantation, the moves by some to initiate clinical trials, and the amount of interest that has been aroused in the subject, an examination of the ethical issues that arise from xenotransplantation is timely. The following principal ethical concerns arising from xenotransplantation were identified by the Working Party and have been discussed in the body of the report:

1 Is using animals to provide organs and tissue for transplantation into human beings acceptable? Are there special concerns about the use of higher primates, or of genetically modified animals (Chapter 4)?

2 If some use of animals for xenotransplantation is considered ethically acceptable, how can the welfare of the animals be adequately protected (Chapter 5)?

3 Xenotransplantation raises the possibility that infectious diseases of animals will be transmitted into the human population. How can this risk be assessed and managed (Chapter 6)?

4 When should clinical trials of xenotransplantation start and how can the welfare and interests of early patients be protected (Chapter 7)?

5 How should the introduction and provision of xenotransplantation, should it develop into a successful clinical treatment, be managed? What are the implications for the financing of the health service if xenotransplantation is successful (Chapter 8)?

6 What attitudes will people have to xenotransplantation and how will individual recipients adjust to receiving a xenograft? What will be the effect of developments in xenotransplantation on the willingness of human beings to donate their organs (Chapter 9)?

10.6 These issues were discussed in the body of the report. The conclusions are summarised below. A series of recommendations is offered to demonstrate how the conclusions should be implemented in practice. The interests at stake and the potential consequences are so great that there is a need for regulation and control of xenotransplantation at a national level. The Working Party recommends an Advisory Committee on Xenotransplantation is established to perform these functions (paragraphs 6.38 - 6.41).

Animal concerns: principles

10.7 Current thinking about the use of animals for medical purposes has been reviewed in Chapter 4. One line of thought holds that when judging whether it is acceptable to use animals for medical purposes, it is necessary to consider whether the pain and suffering of the animals is justified by the potential benefit to human beings (paragraphs 4.5 - 4.6). Another line of thought suggests that animals, like human beings, have rights that must be respected when considering their use for such purposes (paragraphs 4.7 - 4.8). Whether the argument is framed in terms of the interests or the rights of animals, the crucial point is the extent to which animals share the features supposed to be important to human interests and rights. The feature to which most importance has generally been attached is that of self-awareness (paragraph 4.9). To be self-aware requires a high degree of intelligence, the capacity to make comparisons and judgements, and a language with which to articulate them. It has been argued that suffering and death are uniquely painful to a self-aware being who not only senses pain but can also perceive the damage being done to his or her self and future.

10.8 The Working Party accepted that some use of animals for medical purposes is "*an undesirable but unavoidable necessity*" and that "*in the absence of any scientifically and morally acceptable alternative, some use of animals . . . can be justified as necessary to safeguard and improve the heath and alleviate the suffering of human beings*". Not every benefit to human beings will justify the use of animals and, in some cases, the adverse effects on the animals will be so serious as to preclude their use. This conclusion drew on the position set out by the Institute of Medical Ethics towards biomedical research using animals (paragraphs 4.25 - 4.27).

The use of primates for xenotransplantation

10.9 Even if some use of animals for medical purposes can be justified in principle, their use for xenotransplantation raises specific issues that need further consideration. Particular concerns are raised by the use of primates, such as baboons (paragraphs 4.28 - 4.41). The high degree of evolutionary relatedness between human beings and primates both suggests that xenotransplantation of primate organs and tissue might be successful and also raises questions about whether it is ethical to use primates in ways that it is not considered acceptable to use human beings. Certainly, any harm suffered by primates should be given great weight. This position is reflected in the principles underlying current practice in the UK. **The Working Party endorses the special protection afforded to primates used for medical and scientific purposes.**

10.10 The Working Party would accept the use of very small numbers of primates as **recipients of organs** during research to develop xenotransplantation of organs and tissue from non-primates. In this case, using a small number of primates for research, while undesirable, can be justified by the potential benefits if xenotransplantation were to become a successful procedure (paragraph 4.38).

10.11 The routine use of higher primates to supply organs for xenotransplantation on a scale sufficient to meet the organ shortage would represent a new use of primates in the UK. In addition to the special weight given to the harm suffered by primates, other concerns must be taken into account. The endangered status of chimpanzees rules out their use for xenotransplantation. The potential risk of extinction, even to a species like the baboon that is not currently endangered, must be taken seriously. Xenotransplantation using primate organs or tissue may pose particular risks of disease transmission (paragraphs 4.33 - 4.35 and 6.10 - 6.12).

10.12 Given the ethical concerns raised by the use of primates for xenotransplantation, attention has turned to developing the pig as an alternative source of organs and tissue. As discussed below, in the view of the Working Party, the use of pigs for xenotransplantation raises fewer ethical concerns. To develop the use of primates for xenotransplantation, when there is an ethically acceptable alternative, would not be justifiable. **The Working Party recommends that non-primate species should be regarded as the source animals of choice for xenotransplantation.** However, possibilities for alleviating the organ shortage which do not involve the use of animals, such as increased donation of human organs, and the development of artificial organs and tissue, should be actively pursued (paragraph 4.40).

10.13 The Working Party considered the possibility that, after a number of years of research, it might be found that pig organs and tissue could not be used for xenotransplantation. Would it then be ethically acceptable to use primate organs and tissue for xenotransplantation? The members of the Working Party were agreed that the use of primates would be ethically **unacceptable** if **any** of the following conditions obtained:

- improving the supply of human organs and the use of alternative methods of organs replacement such as mechanical organs and tissue replacement could meet the organ shortage;
- the use of higher primates would result in them becoming an endangered species;
- concerns about the possible transmission of disease from higher primates to human beings could not be met; or
- the welfare of the animals could not be maintained to a high standard.

These conditions would rule out all use of chimpanzees on conservation grounds. When considering the hypothetical situation in which the conditions might be satisfied for a species such as the baboon, some members of the Working Party felt that the use of primates to supply organs for xenotransplantation would never be acceptable. Other members of the Working Party felt that, should these circumstances come to prevail, it would be appropriate to reconsider the use of higher primates to supply organs for xenotransplantation (paragraph 4.41).

The use of pigs for xenotransplantation

10.14 While the pig is an animal of sufficient intelligence and sociability to make welfare considerations paramount, there is less evidence that it shares capacities with human beings to the extent that primates do. As such, the adverse effects suffered by the pigs used to supply organs for xenotransplantation would not outweigh the potential benefits to human beings. It is also difficult to see how, in a society in which the breeding of pigs for food and clothing is accepted, their use for life-saving medical procedures such as xenotransplantation could be unacceptable. **The Working Party concluded that the use of pigs for the routine supply of organs for xenotransplantation was ethically acceptable (paragraph 4.42).**

10.15 If pigs are used for xenotransplantation they are likely to have been genetically modified so the human immune response to the pig organs and tissue is reduced. The production of transgenic pigs for xenotransplantation is likely to involve the transfer of a gene or a few genes of human origin. This is a very small and specific change.

It is only in combination with all the other genes that make up the human genome that a particular gene contributes to the specification of the characteristics of the human species. Thus, inserting these genes into a transgenic pig would not destroy the integrity of either species. Species boundaries, in any case, are not inviolable but change through a number of other processes. **The Working Party concluded that the use of transgenic pigs that have been genetically modified to reduce the human immune response to pig organs was ethically acceptable** (paragraphs 4.45 - 4.49). Monitoring the welfare of transgenic animals is discussed below (paragraphs 10.18 - 10.23).

10.16 Should xenotransplantation become widespread, it is possible that surpluses of transgenic pigs may arise, raising the question whether they should be made available on the general agricultural market and used for food. Regulatory mechanisms are in place to examine the acceptability of any proposal to release transgenic animals into the environment or to allow them to enter the food chain (paragraphs 4.50 - 4.52).

10.17 Should the organs and tissue of transgenic pigs be effective for xenotransplantation, applications may be made to patent the pig strains. A detailed discussion of the ethics of patenting transgenic animals lay outside the scope of this report. The issues have been examined in some detail in a previous report of the Nuffield Council on Bioethics, **Human Tissue : Ethical and Legal Issues**, and elsewhere. Proposals to patent transgenic pigs produced for xenotransplantation would increase the debate about the morality and legality of patenting transgenic animals. This adds force to the recommendation of the Nuffield Council in that report "*that the Government joins with other member states of the European Patent Convention (EPC) in adopting a protocol to the EPC which would set out in some detail the criteria to be used by national courts when applying the immorality exclusion to patents in the area of human and animal tissue*" (paragraphs 4.53 - 4.54).

Animal concerns: practice

10.18 In the UK, animals used for scientific purposes are protected by the Animals (Scientific Procedures) Act 1986 (the 1986 Act). Before the use of animals is permitted, the likely adverse effects on the animals must be weighed against the benefits likely to accrue from their use. The Home Office Inspectorate grants licences, in consultation where necessary with the Animal Procedures Committee. The use of animals for xenotransplantation raises questions about their breeding, especially if they are genetically modified, the welfare implications of producing animals free from infectious organisms, and their slaughter. **The Working Party recommends that the convention by which the Animal Procedures Committee advises on project licences in difficult areas should extend to applications for the use of animals for xenotransplantation.** When weighing the harm and the benefits of the use of animals for xenotransplantation, the ethical issues discussed in Chapter 4 should be taken into account (paragraphs 5.2 - 5.5).

10.19 Xenotransplantation research may require the use of limited numbers of primates as xenograft recipients. Primates are afforded special protection by the 1986 Act. Project applications involving primates are examined by the Animal Procedures Committee and the Home Office sets standards for the care and welfare of primates involved in research. The Working Party recommended that non-primate species should be regarded as the source animals of choice for xenotransplantation. What follows, therefore, refers to the welfare implications of the use of non-primate animals, notably transgenic pigs, to supply organs and tissue for xenotransplantation (paragraphs 5.6 - 5.8).

10.20 The breeding of transgenic animals is under the control of the 1986 Act. Transgenic animals can, in principle, be released from the control of the 1986 Act if there is no significant effect on the animals' welfare after two generations. If they are released, welfare concerns would be covered by the less demanding standards regulating agricultural practice and animal husbandry (paragraphs 5.9 - 5.17).

10.21 Animals used to provide organs and tissue will need to be free, as far as possible, from infectious organisms in order to reduce the risk that xenotransplantation will lead to the transmission of diseases into the human population. Repeated testing of animals and other procedures may adversely affect animal welfare. **The Working Party recommends that, when decisions are made about the acceptability of using animals for xenotransplantation, particular attention is paid to reducing the adverse effects associated with the need to produce animals free from infectious organisms** (paragraphs 5.18 - 5.22).

10.22 Removal of organs or tissue from anaesthetised animals will come under the control of the 1986 Act. It is possible, however, that killing animals and removing their organs without the use of an anaesthetic would not come under the control of the 1986 Act. It would be possible, in principle, to remove non-vital organs, or tissues that regenerate, sequentially from animals. This could well result in an increase in animal suffering. The Home Office has stated that the provisions of the 1986 Act regarding re-use of animals would preclude the sequential removal of organs or tissue. **The Working Party recommends that the Animals (Scientific Procedures) Act should continue to be interpreted as prohibiting sequential removal from animals of tissues or organs for transplantation** (paragraphs 5.23 - 5.26).

10.23 Important welfare implications are raised by the breeding of transgenic animals; producing animals free from infectious organisms; and removing organs and tissue from animals for xenotransplantation. There is some uncertainty about whether, in practice, all these aspects would be covered by the 1986 Act. In view of the important welfare implications raised by xenotransplantation, **the Working Party**

recommends that the Home Office should require that all animals used for xenotransplantation are protected under the Animals (Scientific Procedures) Act 1986. Any reputable company producing animals in order to supply organs and tissue for xenotransplantation would, in any case, wish to be licensed under the 1986 Act in order to reassure the public that their activities were meeting the highest standards of animal welfare. **The Working Party recommends that the standards set by the 1986 Act become the minimum for the industry** (paragraph 5.27).

Transmission of infectious diseases

10.24 Xenotransplantation of animal organs and tissue carries with it the potential risk that diseases will be transmitted from animals to xenograft recipients and to the wider human population (Chapter 6). It is difficult to assess this risk, since it is impossible to predict whether infectious organisms that are harmless in their animal host will cause disease in human xenograft recipients or whether the disease will spread into the wider human population. There are certain to be infectious organisms of both primates and pigs that are currently unknown, and some of these might cause disease in human beings. There is evidence that infectious organisms of primates, notably viruses, can pass into the human population and cause disease. This supports the recommendation that non-primate species should be regarded as the source animals of choice for xenotransplantation. The possible risk of disease transmission from pigs, however, also requires careful consideration (paragraphs 6.10 - 6.12).

10.25 It is not possible to predict or quantify the risk that xenotransplantation will result in the emergence of new human diseases. But in the worst case, the consequences could be far-reaching and difficult to control. The principle of precaution requires that action is taken to avoid risks **in advance** of certainty about their nature. It suggests that the burden of proof should lie with those developing the technology to demonstrate that it will not cause serious harm. **The Working Party concluded that the risks associated with possible transmission of infectious diseases as a consequence of xenotransplantation have not been adequately dealt with. It would not be ethical therefore to begin clinical trials of xenotransplantation involving human beings.** In order to address the risks of disease transmission associated with xenotransplantation, the Working Party suggests that the measures set out below should be taken (paragraphs 6.20 - 6.23).

10.26 Stringent efforts should be made to assemble as much information as possible about the risks of disease transmission **before** further xenotransplantation goes ahead. This would involve reviewing existing research and undertaking new research where necessary on the infectious organisms of primates and pigs and the possibility of transmission of disease to human beings. Reliable and accurate methods for identifying potentially dangerous infectious organisms in both source animals and human recipients should be in place before clinical xenotransplantation trials are undertaken (paragraphs 6.24 - 6.26).

10.27 Xenotransplantation should use only source animals reared in conditions in which all known infectious organisms are monitored and controlled. It is ethically unacceptable to use source organs from animals that are known to be infected with infectious organisms (pathogens) which can be eliminated. **The Working Party recommends that a code of practice should be drawn up specifying which organisms should be excluded from specified-pathogen free animals. Xenotransplantation teams should be required to exclude from source animals all the pathogens listed in the code of practice.** Mechanisms should be in place to allow the list of organisms to be updated in the light of experience. The code of practice should recommend the diagnostic tests to be performed by accredited test centres. There is currently no regulatory mechanism that would cover the safety and quality of animal organs and tissue. **The Working Party recommends that a regulatory framework is devised to control the safety and quality of animal organs and tissue for xenotransplantation** (paragraphs 6.27 - 6.32).

10.28 There should be thorough monitoring of early recipients, with regular testing for signs and symptoms of disease. **The Working Party recommends that standards and mechanisms for monitoring xenograft recipients and for the action to be taken in case of disease transmission should be in place before human trials begin. It should be a requirement of clinical trials that the need for monitoring is explained to the patient and that it is made clear that consent to the operation also implies consent to subsequent monitoring** (paragraphs 6.33 - 6.36).

10.29 In order to facilitate the recording and analysis of information concerning possible disease transmission, **the Working Party recommends that xenotransplantation teams should be required to record all information concerning individual xenograft recipients in a xenotransplantation register maintained by an independent body.** Suitably anonymised data should be reviewed for evidence of the possible emergence of new diseases. Since, initially, xenograft recipients are likely to be few, and to be spread across several countries, international co-operation should take place to enable effective review of all the available evidence (paragraph 6.37).

10.30 There should be a commitment to suspend, amend or, if necessary, discontinue xenotransplantation procedures at any signs that new infectious diseases are emerging (paragraph 6.23).

Advisory Committee on Xenotransplantation

10.31 Implementing the precautions outlined above will require an expert and authoritative body that is independent of the research teams at work on xenotransplantation. In view of the seriousness of the issues and of the public concerns about the technique, **the Working Party recommends that the Department of Health should establish an Advisory Committee on Xenotransplantation.** The proposed Advisory Committee on Xenotransplantation should combine the necessary scientific and medical expertise to examine early protocols with broader expertise to ensure that the Committee keeps in mind the wide range of issues raised by xenotransplantation. It should be open and accountable. There would be a need for close liaison between the proposed Advisory Committee and the Animal Procedures Committee (paragraphs 6.38 - 6.41).

Early patients

10.32 Xenotransplants should be offered to human patients only when results using animal recipients suggest that these operations will have a reasonable chance of success. There is currently little consensus within the transplantation community, both in the UK and in the US, as to whether the current data using animal recipients justifies progressing to clinical trials. **The Working Party recommends that no xenotransplantation trials involving human recipients should proceed until the proposed Advisory Committee on Xenotransplantation is in place and has approved the trials** (paragraphs 7.2 - 7.8). The restriction of xenotransplantation to a small number of centres would allow effective control of the risks associated with the potential transmission of infectious diseases and careful protection of early patients (paragraph 7.34).

10.33 Local Research Ethics Committees (LRECs) review, and must approve, all proposals for research involving human participants. All proposals for clinical trials of xenotransplantation will require LREC approval, in addition to the approval of the proposed Advisory Committee on Xenotransplantation (paragraph 7.9).

10.34 Even when the results from animal experiments suggest that xenotransplantation involving human recipients is justifiable, the early clinical trials will involve unknown and unpredictable risks. The question then becomes how best to protect early patients' welfare and interests. It is of the utmost importance that potential patients give free and properly informed consent to participation in the first xenotransplantation trials. **The Working Party recommends that the consent of patients to participation in xenotransplantation trials is sought by appropriately trained professionals who are independent of the xenotransplantation team. The information given to prospective recipients should include an estimation of likely success, attendant risks and subsequent quality of life** (paragraphs 7.14 - 7.18).

Patients consenting to xenotransplantation should be informed that post-operative monitoring for infectious organisms is an integral part of the procedure, and that their consent to the operation includes consent to this monitoring (paragraph 10.28).

10.35 Teams conducting experimental trials on patients are under a scientific and ethical obligation to research and report the subsequent quality of life of recipients. **The Working Party recommends that no protocol to conduct a trial should be accepted unless it contains a commitment to a robust description and assessment of the patient's pre-operative and post-operative quality of life.** Quality of life information should be included in any scientific publication (paragraphs 7.19 - 7.21).

10.36 Special issues arise in the case of children. Xenotransplantation has been proposed as a method of reducing the especially acute shortage of organs for babies and children. Early clinical trials of xenotransplantation will be a form of therapeutic research. Therapeutic research must offer some prospect of genuine benefit for the patient, but it involves greater uncertainties than treatment, and therefore greater caution must be exercised. The British Paediatric Association and the Medical Research Council have advised that therapeutic research should not involve children if it could equally well be performed with adults. It would be difficult to justify the involvement of children in major and risky xenotransplantation trials before some of the uncertainties have been eliminated in trials involving adults. **The Working Party recommends that the first xenotransplantation trials involve adults rather than children** (paragraphs 7.22 - 7.23).

10.37 The special protection afforded children needs to be balanced with the importance of not withholding potentially beneficial treatment, even if that benefit is offered in the context of therapeutic research. If the first adult trials are successful, and there is greater certainty about the benefits, there would be stronger arguments for offering xenotransplantation to children. The question of consent then becomes important. Children between 16 and 18 may be considered capable of consenting on their own behalf to participate in therapeutic research, although a higher level of maturity would probably be required than that needed for consent to medical treatment. Given the complexity of the ethics and law in this area, a cautious approach would be to obtain the consent of the person with parental responsibility before a child under 18 participates in a major procedure like xenotransplantation. The agreement of any child to participation in therapeutic research such as xenotransplantation should always be obtained (paragraph 7.24).

10.38 Similar issues arise for adults who are considered incapable of consenting to participation in therapeutic research because they are mentally incapacitated. The law would appear to be that incapacitated adults may be involved in therapeutic research if this is in their best interests. It would be difficult to justify the involvement of incapacitated adults in the first xenotransplantation trials before some of the major uncertainties have been eliminated in trials involving adults who are capable of weighing the benefits and risks on their own behalf. **The Working Party recommends that the first xenotransplantation trials should not involve adults incapable of consenting to participation on their own behalf** (paragraph 7.25).

10.39 The Medical Research Council has recommended that the participation of incapacitated adults in therapeutic research may be justified if, in addition to evidence that the procedure will benefit the individual, it relates to their incapacitating condition and the relevant knowledge could not be gained by research in adults able to consent. One situation in which this might justify xenotransplantation trials involving the mentally incapacitated is the proposed transplantation of pig fetal neural tissue to treat people suffering from Huntington's disease, a neurodegenerative disorder which affects mental capacity. Such trials should only take place, however, if there is evidence to support progressing from animal research to human trials and to indicate that the procedure will benefit the individuals involved (paragraph 7.26).

10.40 Public policy must be able to take account of different attitudes to xenotransplantation. Some people may wish to refuse xenotransplantation as a form of treatment. If refusing a xenograft reduced a person's priority for a human transplant, consent to xenotransplantation would certainly not be freely given. **The Working Party recommends that, at any stage in the development of xenotransplantation, patients who, for whatever reasons, refuse xenografts should remain entitled to consideration for human organs on the same basis as before their refusal** (paragraphs 7.27 - 7.30).

10.41 What should happen to someone who has accepted a xenograft, but for whom a human organ or tissue at some later date might offer better prospects? In the early stages of development, xenografts are unlikely to be as successful as human transplants, and it is possible that they will only work for a fairly short period of time. **The Working Party recommends that xenograft recipients should remain entitled to consideration for human organ transplantation on the same basis of clinical need as before xenotransplantation.** The Working Party recognises that an implication of this position is that the demand for human organs may not decline, and may even increase, in the early years of xenotransplantation, since xenograft recipients may remain on the waiting list for human organs whereas without a xenograft they might not have survived (paragraph 7.31).

Effects on the health care system

10.42 What are the implications for the NHS, should xenotransplantation move beyond the experimental stage and become a routine surgical procedure? It is likely that the major cost implications of xenotransplantation would arise from the larger number of transplants that would be possible. Should xenotransplantation develop into a successful procedure, decisions about its provision would have to be made within the context of wider debate about resource allocation within the NHS (paragraphs 8.1 - 8.13).

10.43 There are good reasons for introducing new and potentially expensive specialist services in a controlled way. Restricting xenotransplantation to designated centres for the foreseeable future would ensure adequate monitoring of its cost and effectiveness. Already in existence is the Supra Regional Services Advisory Group which is responsible for the introduction and provision of specialist services. **The Working Party recommends that, if xenotransplantation becomes a treatment of choice, the introduction of the treatment into the NHS should be overseen by the Supra Regional Services Advisory Group** (paragraphs 8.14 - 8.17).

Personal and social effects of xenotransplantation

10.44 Attitudes to xenotransplantation will vary. Some may view it as part of a quest to prolong life, in pursuit of which goal, human beings are prepared to abuse their relationship with other animals. Others may regard it as offering a way of providing organs and tissue for transplantation that is preferable to some of the measures proposed for increasing the supply of human organs. There is a need for transparency and openness in the activities of researchers and policy-makers involved in xenotransplantation, and of full debate about its acceptability (paragraphs 9.1 - 9.4).

10.45 It is difficult to predict what the effects of xenotransplantation might be on individual recipients and, in particular, how people's views of their body and of their identity might be affected by xenotransplantation. This highlights the need for more research in this area. **The Working Party recommends that counselling of xenograft recipients should include discussion of the possible personal impact of xenotransplantation. The Working Party further recommends that research should be initiated to assess the personal impact of xenotransplantation on potential and early recipients** (paragraphs 9.5 - 9.15).

10.46 It is highly unlikely that xenotransplantation would eliminate the need for human organs. Xenotransplantation would probably become part of a range of treatments used alongside human organ and tissue transplantation, and the use of artificial substitutes. It is very important to indicate to potential and actual human donors that their gift will be no less precious if it becomes part of the range of available treatments. There is a great responsibility, therefore, on xenotransplant teams, on the media and on those responsible for influencing public opinion to ensure that the reporting of developments in xenotransplantation is as accurate, balanced and unsensational as possible. It should be made clear that, for the foreseeable future, xenotransplantation will not solve the shortage of organs and tissue for transplantation and that there will still be a pressing need for the donation of human organs (paragraphs 9.16 - 9.20).

Implementation of recommendations

10.47 This report has set out the many ethical issues raised by the development of xenotransplantation. In the view of the Working Party, responding to these issues will require the establishment of an Advisory Committee on Xenotransplantation (paragraph 10.31). **The Working Party recommends that the proposed Advisory Committee on Xenotransplantation should produce guidance on best practice and revise that guidance in the light of experience. The responsibilities of the Advisory Committee should include:**

- **assembling and assessing information about the possible risks of disease transmission, and on that basis making recommendations** (paragraph 10.26)
- **establishing a regulatory mechanism to ensure that the appropriate infectious organisms are eliminated from source animals** (paragraph 10.27)
- **developing guidance on the monitoring of future recipients of xenografts and maintaining a register of xenograft recipients** (paragraphs 10.28 - 10.29)
- **approving any xenotransplantation trials involving human recipients and the centres that may undertake such trials** (paragraph 10.32)
- **overseeing issues of consent and conscientious objection** (paragraphs 10.34 - 10.41)
- **assessing the impact of xenotransplantation on individual recipients** (paragraph 10.45)
- **facilitating debate and assessing attitudes to xenotransplantation** (paragraph 10.46).

No xenotransplantation trials involving human recipients should proceed until the proposed Advisory Committee on Xenotransplantation is in place and the above issues have been addressed.

10.48 A particularly wide range of concerns is raised by xenotransplantation, about which people have differing and strongly held views. The Working Party has recommended that the development of xenotransplantation should continue subject to rigorous regulation to ensure protection for potential human recipients and care for animal welfare. Public debate about the ethical issues raised by xenotransplantation will continue. This report is intended to contribute to that debate.

Annex A

Public consultation

1 The Working Party agreed at an early stage that steps should be taken to collect the views of interested parties on xenografts. Early in April 1995 about 130 organisations and individuals were contacted directly and a brief announcement and invitation to comment were carried in the **Daily Telegraph**, **Guardian**, **Independent** and **The Times**. Copies of the letters and information sent out are in Annex B.

2 The list of individuals and organisations contacted is in Annex C. Efforts were made to ensure that the following areas were represented: researchers and practitioners in the field; animal rights and animal welfare organisations; organisations lobbying on genetic engineering; commercial interests and religious groups. It was anticipated that professionals working in the field would alert the Working Party to current scientific developments and issues; other interest groups and members of the public would give a sense of the strength of feeling or indicate themes that might otherwise be missed. The list of submissions received is in Annex D.

3 Most submissions came from organisations or from individuals with an organisational affiliation. The largest group of responses came from universities, colleges, learned societies, research institutes and research councils. The next largest group was that representing religious organisations. Several submissions came from what can be broadly termed animal interest groups. A few submissions came from those with direct commercial interests in this field.

4 The response from members of the public was small. The Working Party received five submissions from individuals writing entirely in their private capacity as concerned citizens and a submission from a group of sixth-formers from Dalriada School, Ballymoney, Northern Ireland. In comments ranging from two or three sentences to half a paragraph, 26 pupils gave their individual reactions to the concept of a xenograft and the possibilities it offers. Almost all the issues discussed in this report were raised in some form across this set of responses. Reactions of amazement and initial doubt amongst these young people gave way, for the most part, to acceptance of something that might benefit humankind - though three responses ruled the idea of xenografts out completely. "*That*", commented one member of the Working Party, "*is as good an indication as any of the range of public opinion in this area.*"

5 The submissions varied considerably. The Working Party is especially grateful for the several specially prepared submissions that were received, running to more than ten, and, in one case, almost forty pages. These represented many hours - sometimes, quite clearly, weeks - of work, and the Working Party is thankful for the public spirit that prompted such extensive effort. Several submissions took the form of a short letter making two or three points relevant to an area discussed in the report, or drawing attention to relevant research, legislation and policy development. Short as these letters were, they were often the result of considerable deliberation and consultation, and the Working Party was much helped by the way in which they gave an overview and a sense of what was at stake. The Working Party also received copies of academic work in progress: chapters from books, excerpts from dissertations, collections of published papers, and copies of articles. This response from specialists in different fields was an immeasurable help to the Working Party.

6 Despite the quality and usefulness of the material that emerged from the consultation, it cannot be taken as a representative indication of public opinion as a whole. The Working Party notes, for example, that the opinions have come more from researchers than from practitioners, and that health workers other than doctors have not responded at all. Interestingly, too, no practising transplant surgeons took the opportunity to express views. A patient perspective emerged very rarely: no patient group responded to the consultation. Beyond this, there are the caveats that often apply to an exercise such as this. The comments are drawn in the main from a more affluent, more educated and more privileged section of the population. Except in so far as the views of some religious leaders represent them, opinions of people from ethnic minority groups remain unexplored. Women's voices are in a small minority among the responses. The sixth-form group gave an important insight into views of young people, but again the bias is towards those from the more privileged sections of the community.

7 The Working Party paid careful attention to the results of the consultation and the submissions were discussed at Working Party meetings. It served as a guide to the range of views that is to be found among interested parties and members of the public. Thus, the public consultation formed an important component of the Working Party's consideration of the issues and the Working Party is grateful to all those who took the trouble to respond.

Annex B

Consultation letters and information pack

Consultation letter to professional bodies

The Nuffield Council on Bioethics is described in the enclosed leaflet. The Council has set up a working party to investigate the issues surrounding the present and proposed uses of animal cells, tissues and organs in the treatment of human disease. I enclose the working party's terms of reference and a list of the members.

The issues raised by this new technology are numerous and include at least: the use and genetic modification of animals in principle; the effects on patients, medical practice and the health care system; and other institutional implications.

I am writing to ask if you wish to comment on any aspect of this study. If so, your comments should be addressed to:

Xenografts
Nuffield Council on Bioethics
28 Bedford Square
London WC1B 3EG

The published report of the study may well include a list of those who have commented. For whatever reason if you wish not to be included in such a list, please make this clear in your comments.

It will be most useful if you let me have your comments in writing by **19 May 1995,** but please do not hesitate to contact me if this will be difficult or if you have any questions,

For the Secretariat of the Working Party on Xenografts

Letter sent to those replying to newspaper advertisements

Thank you for your enquiry.

The issues surrounding the present and proposed uses of animal cells, tissues and organs in the treatment of human disease are numerous, and the Nuffield Council on Bioethics has set up a Working Party to investigate and report on those issues by the end of the year. Part of this process includes gathering public views and the Council would be grateful for any comments that you might like to make.

As background information I have enclosed:

- a leaflet describing the work of the Nuffield Council on Bioethics
- the terms of reference for the study
- some additional guidance from the Council to the Working Party
- a list of the members of the Working Party
- the text of an article from **New Scientist**, *The organ factory of the future*, which is a very readable overview of xenografts.[1]

The published report of the study may well include a list of those who have commented. For whatever reason if you wish not to be included in such a list, please make this clear in your comments. Also it will be helpful if you would identify any special experience that you may have which is relevant to the study.

If you wish to contribute to this present study, it will be most useful if you let me have your comments in writing by **19 May 1995**.

For the Secretariat of the Working Party on Xenografts

1 We are grateful to David Concar and to **New Scientist** for permission to reprint the text of his article for this purpose. The article appeared in **New Scientist**, 18 June 1994, pp 24-9.

Additional guidance from the Nuffield Council on Bioethics

Recent and likely advances

1 The definition of xenografts is potentially wide. If the term, xenograft, is taken to mean the intentional transfer of cells, tissues or organs between species then it would include:

1.1 the transplantation of non-human animal cells, tissues or organs into human beings (non-human animals will subsequently be referred to as animals);
1.2 the transplantation of human cells, tissues or organs into animals; and
1.3 the transplantation of cells, tissues or organs between different species of animals.

2 All these procedures are, or have been, undertaken. An example of the first is the routine and successful use of porcine heart valves in the surgical treatment of patients with heart disease; and, of the second, the insertion of human tissue into immune-deficient mice to explore the pathogenesis of disease.

Definition

3 The wider the definition of tissue then the greater is the scope of xenografts. For the purpose of the Working Party, it is suggested that a xenograft is taken to be the intentional transfer of cells, tissues or organs from animals to humans.

Technical aspects

4 It will be for the Working Party to report fully on the existing technology: what has been done already and what researchers have learned of the difficulties which will need to be overcome if xenografting is to become a safe procedure in the treatment of human illness. Whole organ xenotransplants have been undertaken over the last thirty years using primate donors, but the survival times of the recipients have been very poor: death has occurred usually within days and sometimes within minutes.

5 The human body's reaction to a graft can range from complete acceptance through toleration aided by immunosuppressant drugs to *hyperacute rejection* which is the sudden, extensive and total rejection of the graft. This human immunological response depends on several factors. In very general terms the closer the donor and recipient are genetically, the greater the likelihood of a successful graft: the best case is between identical twins. With a human recipient if the donor is only distantly related in genetic terms then the reaction is likely to be a hyperacute rejection and the graft will fail. One proposed solution to this difficulty is to engineer animals genetically: this would be the creation of transgenic animals as a source of cells, tissues or organs which were more acceptable to the human body. The insertion of human genes into animals is a technique which has already been developed and

researchers have already produced a pig which expressed human Decay Accelerating Factor which is an important step toward avoiding hyperacute rejection.

6 Even with the successful genetic modification of source animals there may be as yet unexplored technical problems with the remaining immunological incompatibilities such as the technique will never prove to be feasible or the effects on humans render it unacceptable.

The need for xenografts

7 The need for xenografts may be seen to arise from a shortfall between the supply and demand for human organs. A recent report stated "*. . . there are not enough organs to meet demand, and the situation is getting worse.*" (**A Question of Give and Take,** King's Fund Institute Research Report 18, Page 15). That report considered ways in which the supply of human organs could be increased. The achievement of health targets, such as those set out in the Government White Paper, **The Health of the Nation**, may reduce but cannot eliminate the overall need arising from, say, heart disorders or renal failure. Meanwhile, advances in surgical techniques and the success of modern immunosuppressants mean that proportionally more patients could be treated with organ transplantation. The supply of cadaveric human organs is falling: improvements in road safety and car design haver significantly reduced the number of accidental deaths. There are doubts that even when supplemented by live donors, organs available are insufficient.

8 In some instances, such as recipients with hepatitis B, the use of an animal rather than a human organ might offer greater chances of survival because the animal organ may be resistant to human specific diseases.

9 The study should also consider the comparative likelihood of the successful development of entirely artificial organs.

Ethical issues and questions

10 The report should consider the likely quality of life which recipients of xenografts might experience. In particular, there is an issue concerning the fate of early recipients, ie those involved at the experimental stage.

11 The report should consider whether there are grounds for the use of different species as potential sources of cells, tissues or organs and, in particular, should consider whether there should be any absolute prohibition on the use of certain species. This will include the ecological impact of such a use and the questions arising from the genetic engineering of those animals.

12 Animals are used by humans for a wide variety of purposes, but mainly as a source of food. This report will consider only the proposed novel and experimental use as a source of cells, tissues or organs for the treatment of human disease and not the use of animals in itself.

13 In the area of animal interests there is a wide spectrum of religious and philosophical views. The study should consider the various ethical frameworks within which a discussion of this novel use of animals can take place meaningfully. In Chapter 11 of **Lives in the Balance: The Report of a Working Party of the Institute of Medical Ethics** (OUP, 1991) the authors state ". . . *there is no shared religious or philosophical world-view which might dictate an agreed answer to the question of how we can adjudicate on conflicts between obligations owed to humanity and to animals.*" However that report achieved a working agreement which was recorded explicitly (it is reproduced in part as Annex A to this paper).[2] Should the need arise, the Working Party on Xenografts will wish to adopt a comparable approach to record the measure of agreement that might be acceptable within the UK.

14 In addition to concerns that genetically engineered animals may suffer "a bad life", there are issues arising from the special conditions under which transgenic donor animals are likely to be bred and kept: for example, will the life of such animals be significantly different from that of farm animals: and if so, what are the likely consequences?

15 Other issues arise from current concerns about the potential risks involved in this new area of research. One example is the transmission of disease (infectious and non-infectious) or of genetic susceptibility to disease across species boundaries, but there may be others: another would be the different biochemical functions of human and animal organs. Such risks should be discussed.

16 The future, successful use of animal cells, tissues or organs in transplant surgery may affect the need and the willingness to give consent to human organ donation.

17 The study should consider the possible effects on communal or social solidarity, most importantly the sharing of the financial risks of ill health, on which most modern health systems are based. Generally, consideration should also be given to the service and financial implications of the widespread adoption of this technology.

Consultation document

18 The study should aim to discover public and professional views by issuing a consultation document.

2 Annex A contained the statement reproduced in paragraph 4.25 of this report.

Annex C

Individuals and organisations contacted

Revd Professor Robin Gill
Dr David King
Revd Dr John Polkinghorne
Professor Margaret Stacey
Association of the British Pharmaceutical Industry
Action of Churches Together in Scotland
Animal Aid
Animal Welfare Foundation
Association of Clinical Cytogeneticists
Association of Medical Research Charities
Association of Community Health Councils for England and Wales
British Medical Association Medical Ethics Committee
Baptist Union
BioIndustry Association
Biotechnology & Biological Sciences Research Council
Bowling Green State University, Ohio: Dept of Philosophy
British Laboratory Animals Veterinary Association
British Organ Donor Society (BODY)
British Paediatric Association
British Union Conference of Seventh-Day Adventists
British Union for the Abolition of Vivisection
British Veterinary Association
Buddhist Society, Centre for Study of Health (CSHSD)
CERES
Catholic Bishops' Committee on Bioethical Issues
Catholic Bishops' Conference of Scotland
Catholic Bishops' Conference of Ireland
Catholic Bishops' Conference of England & Wales
Central Oxford Research Ethics Committee
Centre for Bioethics & Public Policy
Centre for Medical Ethics, Jews' College
Christian Consultative Council for the Welfare of Animals
Christian Medical Fellowship
Church in Wales : Diocese of Monmouth
Church in Wales Centre Board of Mission
Church of England Board for Social Responsibility
Church of Scotland Board for Social Responsibility
Church of Scotland Board of Social Responsibility
Church of Scotland: Society Religion & Technology Project
Clinical Genetics Society
College of Health
Compassion in World Farming
Conference of Medical Royal Colleges

Council of Churches for Britain and Ireland
Department of Health: HEF (Medical)
Department of Health: Mr Edmund Waterhouse
Edinburgh University: Revd Professor Duncan B Forrester
Edinburgh University: Dr R A McCall Smith
Edinburgh University: Professor Neil McIntosh
Edinburgh University: Professor Timothy L S Sprigge
Essex University: Dr W Cartwright
Europe World Society for the Protection of Animals
FRAME
Farm & Food Society
Farm Animal Welfare Coordinating Executive
Genetics Forum
Institute of Health Services Management
Institute of Liver Studies
Institute of Medical Ethics
International Supreme Council of Sikhs
Islamic Cultural Centre
Jain Samaj
Joint Ethico-Medical Committee of Catholic Union of GB and Guild of Catholic Doctors
Joint UK Focus for Biomedical Engineering
King's Fund
Laboratory Animal Science Association
MAFF: Biotechnology Unit
Medical Research Council
Methodist Church Division of Social Responsibility
Monash University, Centre for Human Bioethics: Professor Peter Singer
National Alliance of Women's Organisations
National Anti-vivisection Society
National Consumer Council
National Federation of Women's Institutes
National Spiritual Assembly of the Bahá'ís of the United Kingdom
Nottingham University: B Mepham and C Moore
Office of the Chief Rabbi
Open University: Dr Donna L Dickenson
Patients Association
Presbyterian Church General Secretary
Quaker Concern for Animal Welfare
Quaker Home Service
Royal Society for the Prevention of Cruelty to Animals
Research Defence Society
Royal College of General Practitioners
Royal College of Nursing
Royal College of Obstetricians and Gynaecologists
Royal College of Pathologists
Royal College of Physicians of Edinburgh
Royal College of Physicians & Surgeons of Glasgow
Royal College of Physicians of Ireland

Royal College of Physicians
Royal College of Surgeons in Ireland
Royal College of Surgeons of England
Royal College of Veterinary Surgeons
Royal Society of Edinburgh
Royal Society
Royal Veterinary College
Scottish Society for the Protection of Cruelty to Animals
Sheffield University: Dr J Kinderlerer
Sikh Missionary Society
Society of Ordained Scientists
Soroptimists International
South Buckinghamshire NHS Trust
Surrey University: Professor Ray Spier
Imam of Woking
Townswomen's Guild
Union of Muslim Organisations of UK and Eire
United Kingdom Islamic Mission
United Reformed Church
Universities Federation for Animal Welfare
University of Aberdeen: Revd Professor David Fergusson
University of Birmingham: Liver Research Laboratory
University of Bristol: Professor J E Beringer
University of Brunel: Mr Ian Robinson
University of Cambridge, Centre for Family Research
University of Cambridge: Professor Marilyn Strathern FBA
University of Cambridge: Professor D Broom
University of Cambridge: Mr David White
University of Central Lancashire, Centre for Professional Ethics
University of Colorado at Boulder:Professor Dale Jamieson
University of Copenhagen: Dr Peter Sandoe
University of Keele: Dr Calliope C S Farsides
University of Kent: Professor John Butler
University of Hull: Professor Brenda Almond
University of Lancaster: Dr Sarah Franklin
University of Liverpool: Professor S R L Clark
University of London: Dr R Gillon
University of London: Revd Professor Michael Banner
University of London: Professor John Durant
University of London, UMDS of Guy's and St Thomas's Hospitals: Dr Theresa Marteau
University of Manchester: Professor John Harris
University of Manchester: Professor Margaret Brazier
University of Oxford: Institute of Biological Anthropology
University of Oxford: Mr Michael Lockwood
University of Oxford: Mansfield College
Vegetarian Society
World Society for the Protection of Animals

Annex D

Submissions

Animal Aid
Association of the British Pharmaceutical Industry
Banner M, King's College, University of London (Dept of Theology and Religious Studies)
Barwell L
BioInformation (International) Ltd
Biotechnology & Biological Sciences Research Council
British Biotech
British Laboratory Animals Veterinary Association
British Union for the Abolition of Vivisection
Caddick J, Emmanuel College, University of Cambridge
Centre for Bioethics and Public Policy
Christian Medical Fellowship
Church in Wales
Church of England, Board for Social Responsibility
Church of Scotland, Board of Social Responsibility
Church of Scotland, Working Group on Genetic Engineering in Non-human Life Forms of the Society, Religion and Technology Project
Clark S, University of Liverpool (Dept of Philosophy)
Dalriada School, Ballymoney, N Ireland
Farmers' Forum
Frey R, Bowling Green State University, Ohio (Dept of Philosophy)
Genetics Forum
Gill R, University of Kent
Imutran Ltd
Institute of Medical Ethics
Jain Academy
Joint Ethico-Medical Committee of The Catholic Union of Great Britain and Guild of Catholic Doctors
Levitt M, Centre for Professional Ethics, University of Central Lancashire
Medical Research Council
Mepham B and Moore C, Centre for Applied Bioethics, University of Nottingham
Methodist Church, Division of Social Responsibility
McIntosh N, University of Edinburgh (Dept of Child Life and Health)
McLaughlan A, Bell College of Technology, Hamilton
National Kidney Federation
National Spiritual Assembly of the Bahá'ís of the United Kingdom
Onions D, University of Glasgow (Dept of Veterinary Pathology)
Polkinghorne Revd Professor J, Queen's College, University of Cambridge
PPL Therapeutics
Prowse H
Quaker Concern for Animal Welfare
Reform Synagogues of Great Britain, Medical Ethics Group
Reiss M, Homerton College, Cambridge

Roberts S
Royal College of Obstetricians and Gynaecologists
Royal College of Pathologists
Royal College of Physicians
Royal College of Veterinary Surgeons
Royal Society of Edinburgh
Royal Society for the Prevention of Cruelty to Animals
Silcock S
Skoczylas T
Stacey M, Warwick University
Strathern M, University of Cambridge (Dept of Social Anthropology)
Townswomen's Guild
Union of Muslim Organisations of UK and Eire
Woods T, Brunel University (Centre for the Study of Health)

Annex E

Glossary

α-gal (galactosyl α-1,3-galactose)

α-gal is a sugar molecule found on the surface of pig cells. When pig organs are transplanted into human beings, α-gal acts as an antigen. It is recognised by human antibodies and hyperacute rejection is triggered (paragraph 3.30).

AIDS

The disease AIDS (advanced immunodeficiency syndrome) is caused by the virus HIV (human immunodeficiency virus). The HIV virus infects a type of white blood cells called T-cells and destroys the cell-mediated immune response, leaving the person susceptible to lethal infections. There is normally a latent period of several years between infection with HIV and onset of AIDS (paragraph 6.5)

Antibodies

Antibodies are protein molecules produced by a type of white blood cell called B-cells. Antibodies circulate in the blood and stick to foreign antigens on the cells of foreign organisms or of transplants. This may inactivate the foreign organisms or the transplant directly, or it may enable other white blood cells to destroy them. One important consequence of antibodies sticking to antigens is the activation of a complicated reaction called the complement reaction (paragraphs 3.9 - 3.12)

Antigen

An antigen is a molecule found on the outside of a cell that is recognised as foreign by the immune system. Any infectious organisms entering the body, such as bacteria or viruses, have molecules called antigens on their surface. When the antigens are recognised as foreign, an immune response is mounted to protect the body from infection. Unfortunately, an immune response is also induced by transplantation. This is because the cells of organs and tissues also have antigens on their surface (paragraph 3.10).

Artificial organs

A range of artificial organs and tissues are under development as alternatives to human organ transplantation. These may be totally mechanical devices such as the artificial heart, or they may be bioengineered devices which combine living cells and artificial materials (paragraphs 2.11 - 2.31).

Bacteria

Bacteria are small single-celled infectious organisms. Many are harmless, but some cause diseases. For example, *Mycobacterium tuberculosis* causes tuberculosis.

B-cells

B-cells are the white blood cells that produce antibodies. Antibodies are an important element of the immune response (paragraph 3.9 - 3.11).

Bioengineered organs (see artificial organs)

Brain stem death

Brain stem death is a state in which a person has suffered irreversible brain damage and cannot breathe without the aid of artificial ventilation. It represents the state at which a person becomes truly dead, even though the heart is still beating. There are detailed criteria that enable a reliable diagnosis of brain death to be made. Most organs for transplantation come from people who are brain dead. These people are often called heart-beating donors (paragraph 1.7).

Cadaveric organs

Organs obtained from people who have died (paragraph 1.7)

CD59

CD59 is a human complement regulating molecule. It prevents complement proteins attacking the body's cells. (It is called CD59 because it is a member of a group of cell surface molecules called CD antigens.) (paragraphs 3.13, 3.25 and 3.29).

Cell

The cell is the basic unit of any organism. The human body contains 100 million million cells, each of which is too small to see with the naked eye. Each cell is surrounded by a cell membrane which has, on its surface, protein molecules. Some of these protein molecules are complement regulating proteins. Inside the cell is the nucleus, which contains the genetic material of the cell. Examples of cells are red blood cells, bone marrow cells and pancreatic islet cells. Cells group together to form tissues, and tissues group together to form organs (paragraphs 1.9 and 3.8).

Chromosome

The thread-like DNA in a cell is divided into several separate lengths. Each length forms a structure called a chromosome. There are two copies of each chromosome in every cell. Human cells contain 23 pairs of chromosomes (paragraph 3.28).

Complement proteins (see complement system)

Complement regulating proteins

Complement regulating proteins are molecules found on the surface of the body's cells. They prevent complement proteins attacking the body's cells. Examples of complement regulating proteins are DAF, CD59 and MCP (paragraph 3.12 - 3.13).

Complement system

The complement system is a system of twenty complement proteins found in the blood. It is an important element of the immune response to infectious organisms or to a transplanted organ or tissue. The immune response starts when antibodies stick to antigens on the infectious organism or transplant. A reaction is triggered with one complement protein activating the next, and so on. Ultimately, the complement proteins at the end of the chain attack the foreign organisms or the cells of a transplanted organ, punching holes in them and thus destroying them (paragraph 3.12 - 3.13).

Concordant xenotransplantation

This refers to xenotransplantation between closely related species, where the immune response is not too extreme (paragraph 3.18 - 3.19).

DAF

DAF (decay accelerating factor) is a human complement regulating molecule present on the body's cells. It prevents complement proteins attacking the body's cells (paragraphs 3.13, 3.25 and 3.29).

Dialysis

Dialysis of body fluids is used for patients with kidney failure. A synthetic membrane, or the peritoneum, is used as a dialysing medium across which the blood can be freed of toxic waste products normally excreted by the kidneys. Patients spend several sessions a week having dialysis, and can live relatively normal lives between treatments, which is not the case when most other organs fail (paragraph 2.13).

Discordant xenotransplantation

Xenotransplantation between distantly related species, where the immune response is extreme (paragraph 3.23).

DNA

DNA (deoxyribonucleic acid) is the biochemical substance that genetic material is made of. DNA has a thread-like structure. A gene is a short length of DNA containing the information needed to make one protein. The DNA in a cell is in several long lengths each of which contains many genes. Each length of DNA forms a structure called a chromosome.

Elective ventilation

Elective ventilation involves placing patients for whom death is inevitable on a ventilator so that their breathing is artificially maintained. This keeps their organs in a suitable state for transplantation (paragraph 2.9).

Endogenous retroviruses

Retroviruses are RNA viruses that infect cells and then become inserted into the genetic material of the host cells. Some retroviruses will then start to reproduce. Endogenous retroviruses, however, remain in the genetic material of the host cells in a dormant state. If the retrovirus is inserted into the germ cells (eggs or sperm) it may be passed down from parent to offspring. A procedure such as transplantation might reactivate endogenous retroviruses in a pig organ, leading to the production of new retroviruses in the human recipient and their insertion into the genetic material of the human cells (paragraph 6.9).

Foamy virus

A form of retrovirus that can infect white blood cells (paragraphs 6.10 and 6.28).

Galactosyl α-1,3-galactose (see α-gal)

Gene

A gene is a length of DNA that contains the information needed to make one protein. For example, the haemoglobin gene contains the information needed to make the haemoglobin protein found in red blood cells. The DAF gene contains the information needed to make the complement regulating protein DAF (paragraph 3.25).

Genetic material

Genetic material refers to the material made of DNA in each cell of any organism. The DNA is divided into genes. Each gene contains the information required to produce one protein needed by the cell.

Genetic modification

The process of changing the genetic material of an animal or other organism. The main method of genetically modifying organisms is by transgenesis (paragraphs 3.26 - 3.28 and 4.45 - 49).

Genome

The term genome describes the genetic material of an organism in its entirety, containing a complete set of the information in the DNA.

Heterozygote

Each cell of an organism contains two copies of each gene. In a heterozygote, the two copies are different (paragraph 3.27). Compare homozygote.

Higher primates

Higher primates (more correctly, the simian primates) include all primate species except species such as the loris, bushbaby, ringtail lemur and aye-aye which are known as lower primates (or, more correctly, the prosimian primates) (Figure 4.1).

HIV (see AIDS)

Homozygote

Each cell of an organism contains two copies of each gene. In a homozygote, the two copies are the same (paragraph 3.27). Compare heterozygote.

Hyperacute rejection

Hyperacute rejection is the rapid and strong immune response to a transplanted organ from animals, such as pigs, that are only distantly related to human beings. Within minutes the xenograft is reduced to a black, swollen mass. This is because antibodies attack the pig antigen α-gal (galactosyl α-1,3-galactose). Complement is activated and the cells of the transplanted organ are attacked and destroyed (paragraphs 3.24 and 3.30).

Immunosuppression

This refers to the inhibition of the immune response in order to prevent organ rejection. It is achieved by the use of immunosuppressive drugs which work in a variety of ways (paragraph 3.17).

Islet cells (see pancreatic islet cells)

Live donation

This is when a living person donates an organ or tissue. The most familiar example is blood donation. Kidney donation and bone marrow donation are less common. A very new development is the donation of lung lobes or small bowel. Very occasionally live heart donation can occur, in 'domino' operations, in which a person receiving a heart/lung transplant donates his or her heart for transplantation into someone else (paragraphs 1.7 and 2.6).

Matrix

A matrix is an artificial framework used to support the living cells of a bioengineered organ or tissue. An example is the matrix that is used to support skin cells in order to produce artificial skin (paragraphs 2.30 - 2.31).

MCP

MCP (membrane co-factor protein) is a human complement regulating molecule present on the body's cells. It prevents complement proteins attacking the body's cells (paragraphs 3.13 and 3.25).

Mechanical organs (see artificial organs)

Molecule

Molecules are small particles consisting of groups of atoms. Examples of important biological molecules are proteins and DNA (paragraphs 1.14 and 3.8).

Mutation

A process during which the DNA of an organism changes or mutates. In humans, this can lead to conditions such as cystic fibrosis in which a mutation has occurred in a gene required for proper lung function. The mutant gene is passed down from parent to offspring and so the condition is inherited. In viruses, and other infectious organisms, mutations can lead to the emergence of organisms with new characteristics. In some case they may be more infectious, or cause more serious disease (paragraph 6.9).

Organ

An organ is a structure formed of different types of tissue that performs a particular function. Examples are the kidney, heart, lungs and liver.

Organism

Any living thing, for example, an animal, plant, fungus, bacterium. Viruses and prions are not normally considered to be organisms since they do not show all the characteristics of living things. But, for convenience, in this report, the term organisms was taken to include viruses and prions (paragraph 6.2).

Organ rejection

This refers to the destruction of a transplanted organ due to the immune response of the recipient. The transplanted organ is seen as foreign by the body and so it is attacked by the antibodies and T-cells of the immune system (paragraphs 3.9 - 3.14).

Pancreatic islet cells

The islets of Langerhans are groups of cells found in the pancreas which produce the hormones insulin and glucagon that control blood sugar levels. One cause of diabetes is when the islet cells do not make enough insulin, leading to high levels of blood sugar. Human pancreatic islet cells can be transplanted into patients in order to treat diabetes. Unsuccessful attempts have been made to transplant pig fetal pancreatic islets (Table 3.1).

Patent

A patent is a monopoly right, granted for a limited period, given to an inventor in return for the publication to the world at large of the details of an invention (paragraphs 4.53 - 4.54).

Pathogen

An infectious organism that causes disease (paragraphs 6.29 - 6.30).

Principle of precaution

The principle of precaution offers a method of risk analysis and assessment. It requires that action should be taken to avoid risks in advance of certainty about their nature and suggests that the burden of proof should lie with those developing the technology to demonstrate that it will not cause serious harm (paragraphs 6.20 - 6.23).

Prion

A prion is a small particle made of protein that is thought to cause a type of disease called spongiform encephalopathy. Examples are, in cattle, BSE (bovine spongiform encephalopathy or mad cow disease) and, in human beings, Creutzfeldt-Jakob disease (CJD). The diseases lead to degeneration of the central nervous system. Prions are unusual because they appear to be a unique example of an infectious agent that does not contain genetic material.

Protein

A protein is a particular kind of molecule made up of sub-units called amino-acids. Each cell contains many different kinds of proteins, each with a different function. Muscle cells contain large quantities of two types of protein called actin and myosin (this is why lean meat is a good source of protein). Another example of a protein is DAF, the complement regulating protein found on human cells that stops the immune system attacking the body's own cells. Every protein must be manufactured from the amino-acids that make it up. The information controlling this process is contained in the gene corresponding to that protein. So there is a gene containing the information for the actin protein, and a different gene containing the information for the DAF protein.

Recombination

A form of mutation in which two viruses exchange genetic material, resulting in the production of new viruses, which may have different characteristics (paragraph 6.9.4).

Retrovirus

A type of virus that contains RNA as its genetic material. The HIV virus that causes AIDS is an example of a retrovirus. After a retrovirus has infected a cell, the process of reproduction involves conversion into DNA. The DNA is inserted into the genetic material of the host cell. RNA is then made and used to produce new viruses.

RNA

RNA (ribonucleic acid) is similar to DNA in structure, but it performs a different function in living cells. Certain viruses contain RNA, not DNA. Examples are the virus that causes polio and the HIV virus that causes AIDS. The HIV virus is a particular type of RNA virus called a retrovirus.

Source animal

An animal from which organs or tissue are taken for transplantation into a human being.

Species

A species is a group of individuals that share the same or similar characteristics and which can interbreed to produce fertile offspring.

Specified-pathogen free

The term used to describe an organism from which certain pathogens, or infectious organisms, have been eliminated (paragraphs 6.29 - 6.30).

T-cell

T-cells are white blood cells that produce a cell-mediated immune response. Killer T-cells directly attack cells bearing foreign antigens, ultimately killing them (paragraph 3.14).

Tissue

A tissue is a collection of similar cells that all perform the same function. An example is the neural tissue of the brain. Bone is a type of tissue where the cells are surrounded by hard deposits. Tissues may group together to form organs (paragraph 1.9).

Transgenesis

This refers to the introduction of a foreign gene into an animal or other organism. The transferred gene is called a transgene (paragraphs 3.26 - 3.28 and 4.45 - 4.49).

Transplantation

Transplantation involves the removal of organs, tissue or cells from one organism and their implantation into another organism (paragraph 3.8).

Virus

A minute infectious organism made of genetic material and protein. It is not normally considered to be a living organism, since it cannot live independently. Instead, viruses must infect living cells and reproduce inside them. New virus particles can then leave the cell. In some viruses, such as the herpes viruses, the genetic material is DNA. In others, such as the HIV virus that causes AIDS, the genetic material is a different type, called RNA (paragraph 6.9).

White blood cells

White blood cells (leucocytes) are the blood cells that enable the body to mount an immune response. They are divided into two main groups: B-cells and T-cells (paragraphs 3.9 - 3.14).

Xenotransplantation

Xenotransplantation or xenografting is the transplantation between different species of organs, tissue or cells (paragraph 3.8).

Xenograft

A xenograft is an organ or tissue that has been transplanted from one species into another (paragraph 3.8).

Zoonoses

Zoonoses are animal diseases that can also affect humans (paragraph 6.5).

Acknowledgements

The Working Party wishes to record its thanks to the many professionals and other individuals, too numerous to list here, who have assisted its work.

It is particularly grateful to those individuals and organisations who prepared submissions and for the assistance given by Professor Mildred Blaxter, Dr Heather Draper, Professor Gordon Dunstan, Dr Tony Hope, Professor Robert Lechler, Professor Peter Morris, Professor David Onions and Dr Bob Watt. They all read through an earlier version of the report and we have sought to respond to the insights contained in their detailed comments.

The Working Party would also like to thank Mr Harry Parker for his initial research into the science of xenotransplantation.

Index

Nuffield Council on Bioethics
Publications

Animal-to-Human Transplants : the ethics of xenotransplantation	March 1996	£10.00
Genetic Screening : Ethical Issues	Reprinted May 1995	£7.50
Human Tissue : Ethical and Legal Issues	April 1995	£10.00

To: Mrs Jill Batty, Nuffield Council on Bioethics
28 Bedford Square, London WC1B 3EG, UK
Fax: +44-171-323-4877 Tel: +44-171-631-0566

From: ______________________________

____

____

____

Please send me copy(ies) of
Genetic Screening : Ethical Issues at £7.50 each £ ______

Please send me copy(ies) of
Human Tissue : Ethical and Legal Issues at £10.00 each £ ______

Please send me copy(ies) of **Animal-to-Human Transplants : the ethics of xenotransplantation** at £10.00 each £ ______

Prices include cost of postage within Europe
Please add £2.00 per copy for postage outside Europe £ ______

TOTAL £ ______

I enclose cheque for £ ______ made payable (**in sterling**) to the **Nuffield Foundation**
OR

Please debit my credit card £
Visa/Mastercard/Eurocard no: Expiry date:

______/______/______/______ ______

Name on card ______________________________

Address of cardholder ______________________________

____

____

Postcode ______________________________

Authorised signature ______________________________